I

Copyright © 2004 Lonna Lisa Williams
All rights reserved.

ISBN 1-58898-941-0

I Saw You in the Moon

Lonna Lisa Williams

greatunpublished.com
Title No. 941
2004

I Saw You in the Moon

*I Dedicate this Book
to my family,
to the people of New Zealand,
and to all who have loved the light of the moon
and the One who made it*

*"Points of Light"
By Lonna Lisa Williams*

*When my life is too busy
and exhaustion holds me down
like weights,
I walk outside
into the forest
and look up.*

*Dark trees
like sentinels
encircle the night sky
with stars between their branches
and the wind blows down
from points of light.*

*Cover Photo: The Williams Family at
Lake Pukaki, New Zealand*

Poems by Emily Dickinson

*I'm nobody! Who are you?
Are you nobody, too?
Then there's a pair of us—don't tell!
They'd advertise—you know*

*How dreary to be somebody!
How public like a frog
To tell one's name the livelong day
To an admiring bog!*

*Success is counted sweetest
By those who ne'er succeed.
To comprehend a nectar
Requires sorest need.*

*Not one of all the purple host
Who took the flag to-day
Can tell the definition,
So clear, of victory,*

*As he, defeated, dying,
On whose forbidden ear
The distant strains of triumph
Break, agonized and clear.*

One

Moonlight

I never wanted to write this book. I never wanted to write <u>Crossing the Chemo Room</u>. I didn't care about becoming an expert in anything serious—especially not in an alcoholic childhood, where I was the only one in my family to survive. I didn't want to grow up and learn about divorce, cancer, or miscarriages. I didn't need to know what the words "non-hogkins lymphoma, diffuse cell, intermediate grade" meant.

I prefer fantasy stories and fairy tales. I've been writing those since I was a child—creating amazing new worlds. Nonfiction isn't nearly as much fun as describing slimy gray creatures that lurk in cavepools and wait to jump out at torchbearers who disturb their sleep.

With nonfiction I've got to tell about my own life. I've got to be accurate and do research. And I've got to share my emotions, pouring part of myself into the words. Sometimes I feel that, if I wrote with a pen, the ink would be my own red blood.

"I can't do this, God," I complain when I'm balancing family, housework, homeschool, church, email, website, Internet links, a part-time job at the local paper, and writing my books. "I feel like my nose is glued to the computer screen, and all these facts are bouncing through my head. Surely you could find someone else to write interviews and nonfiction cancer survival stories. Just let me stick to fantasy."

But in my heart I hear the answer,
"I've called you to write your own true story."

I don't always like that answer, and out of frustration I go to The Tolkien Forum (www.thetolkienforum.com), where I'm a member of The Writer's Guild, and post this on my favorite place, The Prancing Pony's Poetry section:

If I had time for poetry
I'd write a line or two
But since I got that newspaper job
My head is full of pooh.

Then I realize that I did manage to write a silly little poem, and I've been thinking about my next fantasy novel. I fall asleep imagining horses that fly over snowy mountains.

The moon wakes me up at midnight, slanting into my window that overlooks the forest. Edd, who has been working hard teaching summer school, snores a little on his side. I slip out of bed and notice how the moonlight touches the new mahogany desk Edd bought me, coating the red wood with a thin plane of white light. The moonlight coats the black laptop and the chair I sit at, and the carpet by my feet. I step out into the plane of moonlight, and it covers my aching, nerve-damaged feet with a silvery beauty for those few seconds that I stand there.

And I look out the window, at the moon shining through the cedar trees, caught partly in their branches, forming patterns on the forest zones of boughs and treetrunks and smaller oaks and manzanitas and uneven ground. The moon touches the stone steps leading up our slope to a path and a single bench by the streambed.

And I think, there is a kind of strange, fantastic beauty in nonfiction.

So I continue to write, drawing from my many journals that I keep on my computer, getting inspiration from God, family, friends, The Internet, music, films, art, books, and—of course—my favorite book, the one that glows in the margins, that has real, life-changing words of power, that brought me through cancer and chemotherapy and countless needles and medical tests: my old blue Bible with its rather worn, silver-edged pages.

And I learn more than I ever wanted to about marketing and book promotion. I've been to a lot of writers' conferences. I even went to the biggest, most prestigious one in Maui. I've conferred with big-time editors and literary agents, who seemed surprised at my body of writing—that I bounce back and forth from science fiction and fantasy to cancer survival stories.

A literary agent at one of these conferences once told me,

"No one will want to read about cancer. It's too depressing."

I sat across the table from him, tears forming in my eyes. I was newly pregnant with what would shortly become my third miscarriage.

"Well, I think you're wrong," I replied in wavering words.

And so he was. My book Crossing the Chemo Room has been read by many cancer patients and their friends and family. I get emails from people all over the world. When I go to buy iced tea at Rite Aid, strangers start up conversations with me about cancer and ask for my book. People who face something like cancer want to see a roadmap through it—drawn by one who has made the journey and survived.

And since my story continues, I will share it with you.

It has been seven years since I finished my chemotherapy treatments. My son Jonathan had his eighth birthday last week. He looks like Frodo from The Lord of the Rings, his wild curly hair and startling blue eyes hobbit-like. His face is almost too beautiful for a boy's, and people often say to me, "He should be a movie star or a model." I reply that I moved to the mountains for a reason, and I don't plan to drive for hours, through traffic, to smoggy Los Angeles.

Sometimes Jonathan tells me he wants to be an actor. He makes me print out the photo of him dressed in his Frodo costume, complete with a maroon vest, green cape, and a simple gold ring hanging from a chain (he won Best Costume at the ice skating rink's contest last fall). He practices signing his autograph. "Frodo" he spells in shaky handwriting across his photograph.

A few minutes later Jonathan insists he'll be a scientist, and he beams from ear to ear as he wears the safety glasses Dad bought for his birthday and examines the glass chemistry set I ordered from Edmund Scientifics. He carries The Periodic Table of Elements chart around as if he knows what all those symbols mean. Once he put a strong magnet next to a Halogen lamp, so that the computer and lamp and fan went off in a big flash as a house fuse blew.

So sometimes we call him Little Frodo, and other times he's Little Mr. Einstein.

He's been taking piano lessons from Andrea Smith whose father Steve has been a music minister for years. Jonathan can read music or "play by ear." When he plays Dad's fancy new keyboard with its variety of sound effects, his hair bounces as he pounds the notes, and he makes up his own songs key by key. Then we call him Little Mozart.

Seven years ago we put him in his bright yellow and blue stroller and pushed him to the back of our valley property, to take our family photo under eucalyptus trees. I wore my short blonde wig, my cheeks still chubby from Prednisone and my face pale.

In that photo, my daughter Jessica was not yet four. Now she is almost eleven, tall for her age, athletic. Her reddish braid dangles past her bottom, and her auburn eyebrows arch expressively over light blue eyes, bird-like, as she tilts her head to kiss her pet parrot whose bright green feathers fan Jessie's cheek—the one with a birthmark shaped like a baby's hand. Jess understands birds, and she wants to be a bird trainer when she grows up. She teaches Penny how to speak and do tricks, then sits for hours at her roll-top desk, carefully drawing bird pictures with her colored pencils:

Scarlet Macaw
Cardinal
Whistling Swan

Canadian Goose
Chickadee

Jessica can walk outside and tell what each songbird sings.

My older children, Kristen and Ryan, are in their early twenties now. Kristen is getting married soon—to a quiet Christian carpenter she met on a mission trip to Mexico (they built houses together for three months). Kristen has her Vocational Nurse's license and works for a big Hospice company in San Diego. She still has long, straight blonde hair, fair blue eyes, and an impish smile. She's great at dressing up in green capes and telling stories in an English accent.

Her brother Ryan, who lifeguards part time and keeps his curly brown hair short, has a dark tan and freckles. He's tall, easy-going, and kind—a good sport with his mom and younger siblings. Never good at keeping quiet, he can say sudden, clever things that surprise most people. He's finishing up his Associate's degree at a junior college and has his Auto Mechanic's certificate. He works for a dealership in San Diego and tries not to let car hoods fall on his neck. He goes to church with his sister and still wonders what plans God has for his life.

We drive down to San Diego to visit Kristen and Ryan, or they journey up the mountain to see us for the weekend.

My husband Edd is a little older but still has his full red beard, blue-green eyes, and bushy brows. He's leading worship music at our local mountain church and teaching college English in the valley. He plays one of his several guitars or his keyboard and sings from the upstairs level of our home, the sound echoing through the evening forest.

He and the children journeyed with me through these past seven years. Part of our journey covered pregnancy loss.

At least forty percent of all pregnancies end in miscarriage, many even before the woman realizes she was pregnant. Way too many end after she gets the good news, tells everyone, and then arrives bleeding in the emergency room. What do you do when your close friend just found out she's having twins next

June, and your own June baby will not even make it past the end of October?

I've had five miscarriages now. I'm an expert. So I sit at my new desk. In between sentences, I stare out the window at the sunlit forest.

Our three-storey mountain house rises into that forest, looking small against the silver Canadian firs and Ponderosa pines that tower above it. It has wood paneling and high windows, decks and fireplaces, and a computer room where we stuff the children's homeschool materials—bookcases, computers, CDs, field guides, rock and feather collections, binoculars, microscopes, solar energy kits, Renoir prints of mothers and babies...

I think of Edd, Jessica, and Jonathan as I sit here and type. They lost five babies too. This last time, almost 2 years ago, Jessica and Jonathan seemed so excited to have a little brother or sister. When they heard the news about my pregnancy, they got out their baby dolls and started dressing them up. When they heard about the miscarriage, they put the dolls away and asked tough questions like:

"Why can't I have a little brother or sister? Couldn't you wait a while and see if the baby would live?"

How could I explain to a six-year-old that a six-week fetus can't live outside its mother's uterus?

I felt like a deflated balloon.

And how does Edd feel? He sat with me for five hours in the emergency room while they did blood tests, exams, and ultrasounds. When the E.R. doctor offered no hope of saving this fetus, Edd turned to me with pain in his eyes and said,

"I'm tired of this. Our last little hope has died."

I could have had my tubes tied and spared myself miscarriages, even though my oncologist told me that I should be able to have more children after chemo if I didn't go into early menopause instead. I could have learned more about joy and peace as I recovered from cancer and chemotherapy. I could have made a conscious choice to go on with my steady life—instead of riding a roller coaster. I could have avoided the thrill and anticipation of finding out I was pregnant followed by the disappointment and pain of losing yet another baby. It seemed as though, just when I was getting over a miscarriage and becoming strong and hopeful again, I got pregnant and had another miscarriage...

I have always done things the hard way.

Besides, I *enjoy* being pregnant—feeling *life* growing inside my body instead of cancer. I'm sure the desire to be pregnant had a lot to do with the cancer. I wanted something amazing to happen after that ordeal. I wanted all my dreams and longings for another child to mean something—to be fulfilled. And how could that possibly happen if I had my tubes tied?

"You're brave," my friend Ann told me once, while we were sitting at the ice rink and watching our children skate. She's an OB-GYN, a baby doctor. She prayed with me before giving me a D & C the year of my fourth miscarriage.

"Brave?" I questioned. "*Stupid* is the word that comes to *my* mind."

"*Brave*," she repeated. "You put yourself in harm's way, risking the possible pain, for a chance at joy. A lot of women, after they've had a miscarriage, stop trying to have a baby."

"Well, after five times, you think I'd take a hint," I replied bitterly. "I've got to stop expecting the impossible and get on with my life. I guess I'll write a book about all this."

"That's a good idea. There's not enough support out there for women who have miscarriages. I could help you do research," she offered.

I stared at her for awhile, not wanting to write this book.

Long after the kids finished skating, Ann's words remained in my mind. They reminded me of what another doctor once said a few months after I finished chemotherapy,

"You must be very brave to have gone through cancer."

I smiled and said nothing though I felt like shouting,

"But I was scared most of the time!"

Maybe that old saying is true: bravery is not the absence of fear, but facing the thing that terrifies you.

So I write nonfiction, even though I'd rather be spinning

another fantasy novel. I find myself weaving my stories through these past seven years, not always in the order they happened. The present mingles with the past and looks toward the future. I hope that my experiences will help someone: maybe even someone who hasn't had alcoholic parents, cancer, or a miscarriage.

When I stand in line at the supermarket and hear someone complain about a broken fingernail, I can't help but smile. I fight back the temptation to say, "I'm a cancer survivor. Here's my card. You can check out my website and read all about it."

My challenges in life have been big. I wish I could have worried only about my fingernails. But, despite everything, I've lived to tell the tale.

Two

Up to the Mountains

I realize that this new book is not just about pregnancy loss. It is a continuation of my cancer survival story. Some people who read <u>Crossing the Chemo Room</u> said that they became so much a part of my world that they were disappointed when my story ended so abruptly. I finished it with a tale about Betty and the lump on her neck. I felt that lump, then looked over my shoulder at the mountains in the distance. I saw the wind blow between Betty and me and wondered if an angel moved in those winter leaves.

Since that night with Betty, over six years have passed. I am still cancer-free. I get to hike in the mountains where Edd moved us four years ago. We got tired of standing in the dusty, over-crowded valley and looking up with longing toward the distant, snow-covered peaks. We came up to the mountains on a vacation and, for fun, decided to look at houses. We ended up buying one. So Edd sacrificed himself to drive an hour each way to work five times a week, up and down mountain roads in snow, fog, rain, or rockslides—roads where several people a year drive off that steep edge and plummet thousands of feet to their deaths.

Edd gave me the mountains. Now the kids and I figure skate at the local rink, swim in the lake, and take long walks in the forest. We find coyotes, bobcats, and bears. Squirrels scamper through interlacing trees. Wildflowers dot the meadows with purple, yellow, and pink. Bees swarm in the lazy air. The setting sun lights up pine trees, all golden at first until the sun slants westward and the rays travel slowly up treetrunks toward the middle and higher branches until it illumines just the tops. Then it jumps off the trees, leaving pink and orange trails in the blue-green western sky. The trees become black against dark blue, until the stars appear—white against a black universe, hanging low and big and bright above us. We feel the cool wind blow down through treetops at the summit. We look over cliffsides toward the millions of lights in the cities below.

And though I am six thousand feet above those cities, I am still tied to them and the stories I left unfinished there.

"The Family on the Computer Screen"

As I recovered from cancer and chemotherapy, my hair started growing back, and my monthly periods resumed. I also felt all the usual post-cancer symptoms like depression, anxiety attacks, guilt for surviving when others do not, sleeplessness, and haunting dreams (what doctors call post-traumatic stress disorder). My symptoms got so bad that I thought something was wrong with my heart, and I ended up in the emergency room and the cardiologist's office. The echocardiogram showed my heart had not been damaged by the chemo.

I learned to reach out—in desperation—to the Internet and the bookstore for information. I called the American Cancer Society and spoke with an oncology nurse. And I joined a cancer support group.

One of my best sources of information was the National Cancer Institute website (http://cancer.nci.nih.gov). There I found helpful articles about the long-term effects of chemo—things an oncologist won't necessarily tell you. One of the articles, called "Facing Forward: Life After Chemotherapy" listed the main long-term effects that I felt even six years after my treatments ended: fatigue, nerve damage, sleeplessness, and chronic pain.

I had been having a rough week. I was tired during the

day, and I couldn't sleep well at night. My feet especially hurt. Ibuprophin did nothing for the pain. Neither did plain Tylenol. My new general practitioner was unwilling to keep prescribing pain medicine, but I knew the pain was not in my mind. I needed to sleep so that I could function the next day as the mother of two active children.

I felt like The Little Mermaid from the original Hans Christian Anderson fairy tale. Unlike the Disney version, when this mermaid becomes human, she must pay a terrible price for her new legs. Each step she takes is agony, like walking on knife blades. She cannot speak to tell her pain. She cannot explain her love and sacrifice to the human prince for whom she left her ocean home. And then the ignorant prince doesn't even pick her. She turns into sea foam at the end of the story, a kind of water angel to guard children from the threatening waves.

That is the price she paid to see a new world.

Tired of being in pain and not sleeping, I got up, went to the upstairs computer room, turned on my Macintosh computer, and searched the National Cancer Institute website until I found the "Facing Forward" article. It listed nerve damage as one of the effects of chemotherapy, and I suddenly realized why my feet hurt.

When I was finishing up my chemo treatments seven years ago, I told the oncology nurse about the numbness in my fingers and toes. To my surprise, she said that the damage was caused by the chemo and would be permanent.

As I stared at my glowing blue computer screen, I read that "neuropathy" is one of the leading causes of pain in post-chemo patients. Doctors, afraid that a patient will become tolerant of or addicted to pain medicine, often will not prescribe it. So the pain goes untreated.

Chemotherapy can even change how your mind works. You may have trouble focusing on a task or remembering things.

Why didn't I know this before? How can the medical profession fill my veins with some of the strongest chemicals known to man and then abandon me when the treatments are done?

Photographs of cancer patients were spread throughout the article, along with these words:

"If I could get over the physical part, if it would stop hurting, I think I would be fine." — Rose, lung cancer survivor, 70.

"I don't think you ever forget the fact that it is always possible for it to come back." — Grant, leukemia survivor, 68.

"As long as I was in treatment, I was killing the cancer. [After treatment] I was waiting for the other shoe to fall." — Judy, breast and thyroid cancer survivor, 45.

"I found myself kind of going through the motions, through the treatments, through the doctor's appointments. I never really stopped to consider the emotional side of things. After I finally realized what I was dealing with, I didn't feel like I had the emotional support I needed." — Carmen, Hodgkin's disease survivor, 20.

"I went [to radiation treatment] every day, and they treated me, and we were like ... family. And now there's this instant separation." — Tom, prostate cancer survivor, 70.

"A process of assessing the 'values' of [my past life] took place. I did not want to stay in the 'sick' world, but my former world seemed so superficial." — Ronnie, colon cancer survivor, 62.

As I scrolled down on my Internet browser, I saw so many photos, so many stories. I stared at the faces on the screen: black or brown or white, male or female, old or young. Tears started pouring down my face as I sat there alone in the computer room at one in the morning.

I live with a loving family. Edd encourages me to write, do research, and help other cancer patients. Jonathan cuddles with me, comforting me somehow for all I've been through. Jessica makes me laugh at the things she says. But none of them have been through cancer, and neither have most of my friends. I haven't gone to a cancer support group since we moved to the mountains.

This is my family, here, on the computer screen, I thought as I wept and touched the cold glass with my numb fingertip. The glass poured out light toward me, as if the lives in the photos touched me back.

∽

I probably should join a cancer support group again. I could fit it into my busy schedule somehow. But sometimes the best support groups are the informal ones that happen through emails or when one cancer survivor visits another:

"Doris' Backpack"

Doris Bowers is our mountain homeschool science teacher. In her sixties, she can still outhike a thirty-year-old fireman on mountain trails. She has known these mountains for over forty years. Go with her on a trip, and she will show you wonders. She will lead you past waterfalls and fern grottos and meadows filled with wildflowers. She will show you where the wild cougars roam through twilight and where the white egrets land on a mountain lake. She will lead you 12,000 feet to the Summit where nothing grows and snow nestles in the cracked gray granite.

Doris wears her whitish hair tied back in a black bow, a white-collared shirt, jeans, and boots. She is a naturalist, primarily a botanist, and her happiest times are leading a group of children through the forest, showing them gray lichen on treetrunks. She can teach oceanography, filling a classroom with seacreatures and ocean photos. She's been to Mount Ararat in Turkey, looking for petrified seashells and Noah's Ark. She studied archeology in Israel. She can conduct a real archeological dig, unearthing bits of pottery and glass bottles from the nineteenth century when loggers settled these mountains. I have a photo of her, kneeling in a mound of dirt, surrounded by children. She stares up at the camera, the sun lighting her face beneath her white Tilly hat.

Doris got breast cancer twenty years ago and survived that. Then, ten years ago, she found melanoma in her leg. She had surgery, and the doctors told her she would not hike a mile again. Undaunted, she left her backpack out in her living room for inspiration, and a year later she was climbing our local mountains. Recently, her melanoma has returned, and this time she had to go into the hospital for more surgery and strong chemotherapy.

I visited her in her mountain home not long after her last treatment. Her hair had thinned a little but not fallen out. She looked a little smaller and paler but still every bit the naturalist, sitting in her log cabin with its stone fireplace and wood mantel decked with photographs, books, and dried plants. Stacked around her were boxes of paperwork and projects: parts of an archeological dig to catalog, seeds to identify, insects to mount, and medical insurance bills to deal with.

For a moment I was a little girl again, sitting with my grandmother the college professor who surrounded herself with her research papers. I felt comforted, as if I had entered a quiet museum full of the familiar and the unexpected.

We talked in calm tones about her recent treatments and side effects and about my long-term struggles after chemo.

"I want to start teaching again," Doris said, a wistful look in her blue eyes. "Just put me in front of a group of children, inside or outside, and I am happy. "

Doris never had a child of her own, but you could not tell by the way she relates with young people.

"I'd also like to hike again," she continued, nodding toward her blue backpack that sat in the corner. "I make myself go out to work in my garden. When I was in the hospital, I could barely walk to the bathroom."

"You'll be hiking again," I assured her. "Let me know when you're going. I would love to hike with you in the mountains."

We continued chatting. It was nice to relax and carry on an uninterrupted adult conversation while Jessica and Jonathan were at camp. When it was time for me to go pick them up, I followed Doris out to her yard. A clump of dried white flowers stood in a ceramic pot.

"Would you like to take these home?" she asked, pointing to the moon-shaped, translucent silver seed pods that dotted dried brown stalks. "These are called moon flowers or lunaria or silver dollar plant."

"Sure," I said, picking up part of the clump.

"I've been taking the brown seeds out of the seed pods," she continued, going back to the house to fetch some for me. "You could plant them in your yard, and in two years you'll have little purple flowers and then these moon pods."

She put a few seeds into an envelope for me and held it out. I took it out of her hand as if receiving treasure.

"Thanks, Doris. We're looking forward to hearing about the new science classes."

"I'll probably do 'Trees' first. I haven't done that in a while."

"Good. We can always learn about how to survive out in the wild, and I love trees. Jessica did really well in the science part of her S.A.T. test, especially biology. She wants to be a bird trainer. Jonathan wants to be an inventor. He has his little laboratory in our backyard, and he enjoys making potions."

"I'd like to teach chemistry soon," Doris remarks.

We look at each other for a moment as sunlight shines down through treebranches and onto our faces. We are both cancer survivors, bearing the scars but still very much alive.

Three

Finishing the Stories

Let me finish the stories I began in <u>Crossing the Chemo Room</u>. Perhaps I'll add a few:

"Betty"

Betty died a few months after I touched that lump on her neck. She switched doctors and took more chemotherapy treatments (as I had suggested). As a result, she got a strange lung disease. She went into a coma and slipped away in the hospital.

Chemotherapy doesn't always cure.

☙

"Lori"

Lori died a few weeks after I finished my chemo treatments. I didn't find this out until months letter when I got an email from her daughter Jackie:

"I just wanted to thank you so much for the beautiful letter you sent to my grandparents. I just received it from them today. Your letter and the book excerpts really touched me.

My mother, Lori, passed away on July 24, 1996. That same day, I had flown back to Cleveland to visit her. I landed in Cleveland at almost nine in the evening. My boyfriend (at that time) and his mother met me at the gate. It wasn't until I was standing by the baggage claim carousel, excited to get home and see my mother, that they told me the news in two simple words: 'she's gone.' I was in such shock. It felt like the wind had been knocked out of me, and a part of my soul ripped out of my body. My mother was my very best friend. She was my counselor, my confidante, one of the only people in the world that I would ever so willingly give my life for.

When she left for Cleveland, everything was so rushed, because they had to get her on the airplane in a special wheelchair. I only had a few minutes to spend with her, and I never really got to say goodbye—at least not the way that I wanted to. To make matters worse, I had delayed my trip to Cleveland by a few days because the store where I worked was having an inventory count. As a shift supervisor, I felt that I needed to be there. I learned a lesson...work is never so important that it should come before your family. You can always find a new job, but family can never be replaced.

My life today is occupied mostly by school and work. I am a psychology major at a university. I believe that I am still picking up the pieces, both emotionally and financially.

I find that sometimes, I almost forget what has happened. Please understand that I lived away from Mom for over four years. I sometimes think that she's just far away. But then, something wonderful, or something terrible, will happen, and I want to talk to her. I could pick up the phone and dial her old number, but she'll never answer. I won't get to see her sitting at my wedding, she can't give me advice, she'll never get to meet my new boyfriend. Some days, I feel like I've lived through what others see over the course of a full lifetime. But I have grown up stronger, wiser, and more courageous because of it. As my mother would say, I'm 20 going on 45.

You may never understand how much it means to me that my mother touched your life as she did, even if only for a brief time. We've had our rough times, of course, but I have always looked up to her. I know now that she will always be with me. Like the precious angel that she was in my life, she is now an angel for the world."

Linda Biehl died a year after my book ended, just after Christmas, from pneumonia. Her husband John gave me photos to put in my book. Here is my memorial for Linda:

"Linda's Rose"

Today we go to the college to visit Daddy at work. After playing hide and seek for awhile under Daddy's desk, the children ask if they can go outside in the sunlight. Edd leaves to teach, so I take them to the rose garden in front of the Humanities Building. They start climbing on the concrete circle that surrounds the roses. I stoop to smell a huge orange and yellow rose and notice someone walk past me.

"John Biehl?" I ask, standing.

He stares at me, his blue eyes squinting beneath his clear glasses. He looks older, his hair grayer and more wispy about his head.

His wife Linda died early this year, of pneumonia—a complication of chemo treatment, two years after she had a bone marrow transplant for non-hodgkins lymphoma.

"I'm Lonna Williams," I say, holding out my hand.

"Oh, Lonna, I didn't recognize you. You look great!" He smiles and takes my hand.

"Thanks. I was sorry to hear about Linda. You must miss her a lot."

Dumb statement, I think as John lowers his head.

"That sun is so bright—the curse of being fair-skinned and blue-eyed," he mumbles.

"Yeah, I know what you mean. That's why I wear dark sunglasses—and probably why you didn't recognize me. Plus, my hair is different," I lamely reply, holding on to a strand of my curls. We wait a moment in awkward silence.

"Oh, I'm doing all right," he finally offers. "A lot of things came together for Linda her last two years of life, though those two years were hard on her. Her funeral was really beautiful. All her family were there, and kids from her class at school."

"She told me she was a Christian," I mention. John lowers his eyes toward the garden, and I wonder if he sees Linda in a white rose.

"Yes, that was a very important part of who she was."

Our moment of silence is interrupted by Jonathan who picks a rose and brings it to me.

"You shouldn't pick those," I admonish, putting it back in the planter. Jessica pushes Jonathan, who screams and pushes her back.

"I guess I'd better be going," I announce, grabbing Jonathan by the arm.

"Yeah, I've got a biology class to teach." John tips his head in farewell and walks toward the Humanities Building, his shoulders a little stooped and his briefcase heavy in one hand.

Since I finished <u>Crossing the Chemo Room</u>, I've met many other cancer patients. One of them was Vicki, who battled melanoma for years. She died a couple of years ago—at home, peaceful, surrounded by her children. I wrote this for Vicki:

"Dream of Vicki"

I dream of Vicki. She is my age and dying of melanoma. In my dream I visit her in a mountain cabin surrounded by pine trees. Sunlight shines through the window into the wood-panneled room.

"Hello, Lonna," she says from a corner.

Her grayish brown hair hangs down her back, straight and wispy. Her brown eyes shine dark against her pale cheeks.

"I'm glad you finally came to see me. Don't be afraid. I have a present for you."

She gets up from her recliner, takes some red, high-heeled shoes out of a box, and hands them to me.

"They're good for dancing," she sings as she raises her arms above her head. She dances through the cabin and out the open door.

❦

Another friend of mine from our old valley church, the older woman who used to come and "babysit" me the day after my chemo treatments, found out she had carcinoma—and a few weeks later, she died:

"Ramona"

I haven't visited Ramona since last June. I make mental excuses like I've got my hands full with my own two children and their three cousins who are living with us.

The real reason is my own weakness.

I don't want to see Ramona as the cancer progresses. It ravages her body, thins her hair, and fills her with pain. She can barely get up to go to the bathroom. Some days she doesn't get up at all.

I thought I was strong and could bear all this...It's been too soon since I saw Vicki suffer, since I watched Lori decline, since I faced my own cancer.

Murlie, Ramona's daughter, told me that Ramona has been feeling depressed. She wants people to call her on the phone and visit more often.

So today I call Murlie and tell her I'm bringing Linda and Jessica to visit.

We pack some soy-protein bars, Fig Newtons, and my cordless headset phone (Murlie mentioned that Ramona's arm hurts when she holds a receiver). We arrive at Ramona's trailer after dark.

Murlie's eyes have dark, puffy circles under them. Her mouth-corners tense as she greets us. She escorts us through the cluttered trailer and to the back bedroom where her mother lies. Ramona looks pale—almost gray, her bad shoulder and elbow sticking up at an odd angle above the sheets.

She smiles and sits up when the little girls run to hug her. Jessica sets the box of Fig Newtons on the T.V. tray next to Ramona's bed. Linda hands Ramona a protein bar. I report about the church and the people who go there—a place and friends that have so long been Ramona's life. I start to describe the Sunday School room where she taught for years, where she taught Jessie and Linda, which she decorated with Bible verses on patchwork quilts and animal faces...but I pause halfway through because someone else teaches there now, and Ramona cannot do her work for the Lord.

"Thanks for teaching Sunday School all those years," I say awkwardly. I'm not sure if Ramona hears me.

Murlie comes to hand Ramona a paper cup filled with multi-colored pills. Ramona surprises me by swallowing them in one gulp. Murlie holds a straw to Ramona's lips, so she can drink water from a plastic cup and wash the pills down.

Suddenly I see myself a few years ago, walking drowsily through my house—in my green robe, a pink cotton cap covering my hairless head, my hand holding a yellow bowl. Ramona, who has come again to babysit me the day after chemo, hands me a cup of water and my Prednisone pill...

Murlie goes back to the kitchen to wash dishes. As Ramona talks to Jessie and Linda, my eyes wander about her small bedroom. Books, stuffed animals, unused clothes, and Bible verses decorate the room. A verse from a hymn, painted on glass with red flowers, says:

"Because He lives,
I can face tomorrow."

Light emanates from the corners of this room.

"What a lovely clock," I say, picking up the brass and glass timepiece that rests on a shelf above Ramona's bed.

"The home care association gave that to me when I retired," she tells me. I trace her name engraved in cursive letters.

I find it hard to look at Ramona. She's so different now. Her body is shrinking in on itself...

"That's a bright painting," I point to a back-lit gazebo surrounded by pastel flowers.

I SAW YOU IN THE MOON

"It's a Thomas Kinkaid," Ramona tells me. "My children keep buying his art for me."

Ramona's room seems like a portal to another world, as if the window above her bed will melt away to the shores of a glass sea spreading beneath stars—toward a transparent-walled Jerusalem.

Ramona's world is more than our small country church, than her three children and their families, than this trailer filled with objects she collected over a lifetime.

The room and Ramona's connection to another world close in on me. I glance at my watch.

"It's getting late. I'd better get the girls home," I say, leaning over the white-sheeted bed to hug Ramona. Her fragile bones almost burn my fingertips with shared pain. As I pull back, I imagine her with a new body—tall and straight, clothed with light like folds of silk, her face glowing.

Lord, please don't let Ramona suffer much longer, I cry silently.

"Thanks for coming to visit me," she says, her voice low so that I have to lean near her to catch the words.

I wish I had come more often.

The cool night air greets us. Linda points to the cirrus clouds that form a white, patchy quilt above us. The full moon, circled by a yellow halo, shines through the opaque layer.

"What does that mean?" Jessica asks, pointing to the strange moon.

"It means a change is coming," I reply, thinking that more than weather will transform.

Ramona died two days later.

༄

Edd's college colleague and friend Ed Henry died of bone cancer. When we visited him a few weeks before his death, this is what we saw:

"A Better Mountain"

Our friend Ed Henry is dying of bone cancer. Today, on a hot summer day before the Fourth of July, we drive down our mountain to visit him and his family.

We stop at Costco on the way. It's crowded with sweating people getting ready for the holiday. We stock our cart full of summer food—roasted chicken, potato salad, watermelon. We add cranberry juice for Ed who has a catheter.

Traffic isn't bad on this side of the freeway, since everyone seems to be getting away from the city. We exit and find the Henry's quiet suburban neighborhood backed up against dry brown hills.

Melinda, Ed's youngest child, answers the door. She is eight—Jessica's age. She squeals when she sees her old friend.

We haven't seen the Henrys in the two years since we moved to the mountains.

I find Linda in the kitchen. We often talk to each other on the phone, so it doesn't seem that long since I've seen her. She looks pretty much the same—tall, slender, with short black hair, smooth dark brown skin, and glasses. She's wearing jeans and a t-shirt, practical clothing.

She's from Saint Lucia. Ed is from another Caribbean island—Jamaica.

He's lying in the computer room-turned-sick room. Propped up with several pillows on his hospital bed, he looks smaller than I remember. His skin seems darker than ever, a rich chocolate black against the white sheets. He's wearing a hospital gown so that I can see how thin his legs are, with ridges along the shin bones. His feet are wrapped in blue foam. He's paralyzed from the waist down now, and he can't move his right arm.

But he's completely alert. I expected him to be asleep or in a morphine haze.

He shakes my hand with his left arm. His deep brown eyes have black circles around them. On the top left side of his bald head is a lump like a lone horn growing. It's a tumor.

"Hello, Lonna!" he says enthusiastically. I sit down in the

chair next to him. Everyone else is busy with food, so Ed and I are alone in the small room lined with bookshelves.

"How are you doing?" he asks. I look sideways at his eyes and think that the irises look the same as always.

For a moment I see him as I first met him seven years ago. He hired me to teach English part-time at the college. He made me feel at ease during the interview as he sat in a chair by the window, smiling, wearing a brown suit and blue tie.

Ed smiles at me now, and I think that he still looks, in a way, beautiful.

"I'm fine," I reply.

"I read your book. How nice that you got it published. It was good to see it in its finished form. I felt close to it, especially since I read it as a manuscript."

He still sounds like a college professor.

"I feel badly that I didn't finish my book," he admits. I remember how he showed me the first few chapters, typed on neat white pages. "I should have worked on it when the cancer was not so strong in me, when I could still get around."

"Well, you still had the disease," I try to comfort him. "The reason I could finish my book is because the cancer left me."

Ed nods his head a little. I look around the room. Posters of Jamaica adorn the wall, between bookshelves—green cliffs reaching down to teal-colored water, palm trees against a sunset, hills above a jungle.

"How is your home in the mountains?" he asks, and I look back at him. "I meant to come visit you. I think I dreamed of it. It's all made of wood, isn't it?"

"Yes. I described it to you once, over the phone." I pause, trying to create a picture with words, like a 3D image hovering in the air of his sick room.

"I love my mountain home. It has three levels. Downstairs is the spare bedroom, the den, and a bathroom with a tile floor and a huge, walk-in shower. We usually stay on the middle floor with its small kitchen and dining area, living room, and stone fireplace. In the back are the two bedrooms and small bathroom. Upstairs is the loft with a wood rail all along it. But the most wonderful part of the home is the high ceiling made of pine panels—warm, honey-colored wood—with a single long beam at the A-frame top.

"And there's a window three stories tall. It looks out over the upper deck. At dusk you can walk out on that deck. The sky turns dark blue above the horizon of tall evergreens. The moon comes up and shines upon the trees, casting shadows on the slope below. The stars appear, bright and large and low. The wind picks up and blows against your face. You smell a cedar tree and reach out your hand to stroke its scaly green branches. On that deck, you feel like you're in a treehouse."

Ed Henry has closed his eyes. I see a tear in the corner of one of them.

I think he must be wishing he had made it up the mountain.

"We should have come here to see you sooner," I say, touching his arm tentatively. "Maybe I have tired you with all my chatter."

"You haven't tired me. Later, my sleep will be restful. And don't feel badly about not coming before. This was the time. I can understand why you wouldn't want to leave your mountain," he replies, his voice low. He has seen my pretty picture and longs for it.

I feel tears in the back of my throat and wonder again why I survived cancer.

"Thank you," Ed Henry says, reading the look in my eyes.

I think I know why I survived.

Edd comes in with his sheet music and guitar, followed by the three Henry children and our two. Linda waits by the door, and I get up to help her with dinner. We stay and visit for a few hours, Edd playing music in the sickroom and bending down to pray with his old friend.

When we finally leave at nine o'clock, the hot summer day has cooled under darkness and a layer of clouds. The California freeways are not crowded as we head back toward our mountain, past billboards and neon lights and tall buildings. We exit the freeway and climb the familiar curves of our mountain highway.

We reach the five thousand foot level. Above, the nearly full moon breaks out of stormclouds, lining their edges with bright light. I look down, again, at the wide, crowded valley below, filled with a million small lights. Then I look ahead at the darkness lined with trees and a few brave stars. I smile in the darkness and think,

Soon Ed Henry will see a better mountain.

∽

Let me end this chapter with the story of one who survived:

"Josh"

A sixteen-year-old boy named Josh got a rare form of lymphoma in his spine. Josh is the son of our email friend Herb in Texas (a Lutheran minister). The insidious tumor wrapped around Josh's vertebrae and broke it. Josh had terrible pains in his back and thought he'd injured it playing football. Then his doctor discovered the cancer.

Josh spent a lot of time in the hospital, getting a worse form of chemo than I got. Josh almost died. After his last chemo treatment, he swelled up, as Herb put it in an email, "like a pillow with legs." He was battling an infection in his intestines (chemo can wipe out your immune system as well as your cancer). Amazingly, he slowly rallied. After several weeks in the hospital, he was released to go (of all things) dove hunting. In an email from Herb, I read these words:

"We drove out to Luther Hill's pasture-land and unloaded by the windmill which I accidentally shot last year. They don't let one forget such things easily in West Texas. Ruins of old cattle pens stand by the windmill, and the overflow forms a small pond surrounded by three gnarly trees. Josh found a spot under the northeast tree and set up one of the folding chairs and sat down...For the first hour we saw almost no birds, yet the mild and quiet evening surrounded us. I quickly noticed how Ben and Elise chattered with Josh under the tree. How wonderful it was to hear them enjoying one another. Their lost brother was finally among them again.

"Though the doctors thought Josh wouldn't have the strength to fire a gun, he dropped a dove near the windmill."

Four

City of Hope

City of Hope in California is one of the world's top cancer research and treatment facilities, known especially for their work with bone marrow transplants. Sometimes a BMT is the last possible treatment for cancer patients. Two years after the end of my own chemo treatments, I visited a friend at City of Hope:

"Dalilah"

We follow the map I downloaded from the City of Hope website. Twilight falls as we find a long driveway, bordered by trees and white lights, that leads to a gate. A security guard directs us to Hope Village, where Dalilah is staying with her caregiver in Room 42.

Edd drives to the circle at the hospital's main entrance, then turns right past a Japanese garden, a tree-shaded park, a visitor center, and a synagogue. We find Hope Village, park the car, and get out to walk.

Jessica and Jonathan prance toward flowers whose colors are still visible in the half-light: orange, yellow, pink, and purple California poppies.

"They're my favorite!" Jessie exclaims.

We walk on a sidewalk toward the cottages. A woman with a shoulder-length blonde wig sits behind a window. She's typing on a laptop.

That could be me...

We look at numbers. Forty-two is vacant, the beds made.

"She must be at the hospital," I say, turning to Edd who holds Jonathan's hand behind me. "Could we walk from here?"

"Sure," Edd says. We stroll down the sidewalks of this parklike place. The hospital itself looks modern, multi-storied, solidly built. I hesitate before the glass doors of the entryway, reading the metal letters that scroll above me:

City of Hope
National Medical Center
and Beckman Research Institute

I stand on the threshold of a great place—the front line of battle against cancer.

City of Hope began in 1913, at the base of the San Gabriel Mountains, when working-class people erected tents as a refuge for people suffering from tuberculosis. After tuberculosis was cured, cancer became the primary focus. People who cannot afford treatment can get it here for free. City of Hope's philosophy is "there is no profit in curing the body if in the process we destroy the soul." Their thirteen-point creed stresses "the sacredness of man, formed in God's image," "we are our brother's keeper," and "'love thy neighbor as thyself.'" They try to meet the spiritual as well as physical needs of their patients.

Here the first bone marrow transplants were performed in 1976—thousands done since then. Here Linda Biehl had her own bone marrow transplant. Here Linda Biehl died.

Do these glass doors open to eternity, a gateway, like the dream Jacob had in the wilderness when he saw angels ascending and descending on a ladder that bridged earth and Heaven?

As if reading my thoughts, Edd opens the door for me and says,

"I'll bet John Biehl walked through these doors a few times."

The receptionist guides us down long corridors to Urgent

Care which takes us to the BMO (Bone Marrow Oncology) ward. The nurse on duty at Wing Six tells us that Dalilah was admitted to the hospital because of mouth sores. "She's down the hall, in Room 626."

I start ahead of Edd and the kids. The long beige hallway, windowless and lit by panels of fluorescent lights, suddenly closes in around me. My feet don't want to walk down the polished linoleum floor. With each step I think,

I could be in that room at the end of this hall.

Another nurse explains that the children cannot enter Dalilah's room, but they can wait with Edd in the hall. She shows me how to scrub my arms and hands for three minutes and then put on the face mask. Dalilah has already had the strong chemo, and the doctors have already put her bone marrow stem cells back in her system. She can't afford to catch an illness while her blood replenishes itself.

I see her reclining on her bed. The T.V. is on. Her sister-in-law, a shy woman who speaks only Spanish, sits in a chair next to her and watches me. She's also wearing a face mask.

"Hi, Dalilah," I say. "It's Lonna."

Dalilah is wearing a blue knit stocking cap and a hospital gown. Her color is good—not pale. She smiles, her petite face and dark eyes looking very much alive.

"Oh, Lonna," she says in a weak voice. "I'm so glad you came."

I ask how she feels, and she struggles to answer me, swallowing often,

"The mouth sores hurt, and my throat, too."

As I watch Dalilah, I remember the sore mouth and throat I had during chemo. Empathy is a good thing, but I need to learn how to handle it. I wince in pain and blink away the tears. Behind me, Jessica and Jonathan whisper to each other and stare through the open door. I can feel Edd's eyes on my back.

"Don't you be afraid, Lonna. We will beat this cancer. Yours won't come back. I read your story, about your life. God will bless you so much more now to make up for all that you had to suffer. We will live to be old ladies together, you and me. God will send His angels to watch over us."

"I came here to comfort you, and you encourage me," I reply, smiling. "I don't want you to talk too much. Let me read for you."

I read from Romans Chapter Eight:

"What then shall we say to these things?
If God is for us, who can be against us?
He who did not spare His own Son,
but delivered Him up for us all,
how shall He not with Him also
freely give us all things?...

Who shall separate us from the
love of Christ?
Shall tribulation, or distress,
or persecution, or famine,
or nakedness, or peril, or sword?...

Yet in all these things we are
more than conquerors
through Him who loved us,

For I am persuaded that neither death
nor life nor angels nor principalities
nor things present nor things to come,
nor height nor depth,
nor any other created thing,
shall be able to separate us
from the love of God
which is in Christ Jesus our Lord."

After I speak the last word, silence falls for a moment. Then I say a prayer. When I open my eyes I notice a small plastic angel—in a nurse's uniform—pinned to Dalilah's hospital gown, above the area where she first found her cancer.

"Tell Edd thanks for bringing you here," Dalilah says.

I remind her that I'll call to see how she's doing.

"You'll be home with your husband and children soon," I add. "Our two six-year-old girls will play together. You live by Costco, so I'll come see you often!"

Dalilah laughs and places a hand to her throat. I turn around and find Edd and the children waiting.

"Thanks for coming here with me," I say to Edd as I grab his arm and walk through a series of long hallways toward the hospital entrance. Jessica and Jonathan skip along next to us. "I didn't want to come here alone."

We see a boy of about seven years old walking toward us with his parents. He's wearing a small hospital gown and a face mask. He has no hair.

"I'm glad I came with you," Edd replies. We stop to get Kit Kats and soda from a vending machine, and I pick up some free brochures.

Glass doors open to the chilly evening. Edd and I sit down on a bench under a flowering tree. Jessica and Jonathan chase each other in circles around a large fountain. In the middle of the fountain rises—toward the starry night—a bronze statue of a man and a woman, dancing and holding a baby high between them. Edd and I look into each other's eyes.

"Come," he says, standing and taking my hand. "It's time to go home."

⁂

Dalilah recovered from her bone marrow transplant and, five years later, still sends me Christmas cards.

I first met Dalilah in the valley, at a breast cancer support group. We were a lively bunch. Here is my first experience with them:

"Dalilah's List"

The "Young Women's Breast Cancer Support Group"

meets at Dr. Schinke's office on the first Tuesday evening of each month. I figure I'm qualified to join this group because I had cancer in my breast.

Seven of us "survivors" gather in a circle in the office waiting room. We are diverse—dark-haired and petite, large and blonde, Asian or Mexican or white. A couple of the women wear pink enameled ribbon pins. We take turns telling our cancer stories. Only one other woman had a lumpectomy—all the rest had at least one breast and some lymph nodes removed. Some had chemo, some radiation, and some both. I didn't realize there were so many types of breast cancer.

Lori, the leader, candidly and humorously relates her children's reaction to her reconstructive surgery.

"When I wore a swimsuit this summer, my eleven-year-old son kept saying, 'Mom, put it back in.'" He didn't want anyone to see the scars."

We giggle.

"But, heck," Lori continues, "my breasts and my hair were always the two things I liked best about my body, and the cancer took away both."

It has been three years since her treatment. She tosses her long blonde hair, and from where I am sitting, I can not tell that one of her breasts was reconstructed. With her body type and personality, she reminds me of another Lori...

A latecomer to our group, Delilah, sits shyly next to her husband and every so often wipes tears from her eyes. A petite Mexican-American in her early thirties, she wears a short blonde wig which reminds me of the one I used to wear. She was recently diagnosed and does not understand exactly what kind of breast cancer she has or how it will be treated. Her husband, looking uncomfortable, murmurs something about picking Delilah up later—and leaves the office.

After sharing breast woes, we talk about husbands.

"When I was going through chemo, I was mad at my husband," I confess. "I blamed him for my cancer, and I thought he could have helped me more somehow. He seemed to withdraw from me..."

"It's common for husbands to withdraw from their wives who have breast cancer," Lori informs us.

"My boyfriend didn't want to make my depression worse by joining in," Renee says. An elegant Asian woman, she wears a brass-buttoned navy suit. "He thought that if he ignored it, it would go away."

"Well, my man and I are still close," Jeanne giggles. She shows us her quarter-inch hair under a baseball cap. "We go out for steak dinner, have a little wine, and then go home and snuggle."

"You eat red meat, drink, and have sex?" Delilah asks, amazed. "I've been avoiding fatty foods and alcohol. And I'm afraid to get close to my husband..."

Jeanne borrows my little notebook and writes out a prescription for Delilah to giver her husband:

1. Hamburger
2. Margarita
3. Sex

Delilah blushes and smiles tentatively, a tissue still held in one hand.

After Delilah leaves early because of her three children waiting at home, Lori explains to us that when Delilah's family visited from Mexico, they wouldn't sit next to her for fear of catching cancer.

"'She's going to die,' her sisters whispered to their children. Can you imagine what this woman is up against?" Lori asks us.

I ask the group if they experienced anxiety attacks or post-traumatic stress disorder. Kim (who has been mostly quiet) turns to me and admits,

"I still have nightmares about the cancer returning. My treatment ended just over a year ago. I was so afraid that the cancer would return that I was feeling my breasts all the time."

We all nod our heads, understanding.

"I'm lucky I had just a lumpectomy. I'm trying not to hate

or fear my breasts but be glad to still have them. I've come up with a plan to do a breast exam only once a month—to cut down on the paranoia," Kim continues.

Her long dark hair (she didn't get chemo) half hides her face as she speaks, yet I can see her hazel eyes under their lashes.

Lori shares news on upcoming breast cancer events, and I decide I'll come back to this group.

Another meeting went like this:

"H.O.P.E."

Before our group gets officially started, an elderly man walks in to tell us that his wife died of cancer.

"Oh, I thought this was the other group," he says shyly, his shoulders stooped a little.

"You must be thinking about the H.O.P.E. (Helping Other People Emotionally) group that meets on Wednesday nights," Lori, our leader, gently informs him. "That group is for any type of cancer. This is for breast cancer."

"Yes, I guess it did meet on Wednesday nights. They were such a help to Mary, and I wanted to let them know about her passing. Since she left, I've been bad about keeping my calendar straight..." he drifts off, lowering his eyes. "Anyway, sorry to bother you," he adds as he puts his hat back on and starts to leave.

"We're sorry about your loss," Lori says in a low voice. She and I look at each other as the man walks out of sight, down the hallway toward the radiation room and the back exit.

"Poor man," she comments. Our group stays silent for a moment.

Then Wendy, wearing a blonde wig instead of a dark one, tells us how she singed the bangs on her other wig while she was baking cookies.

"You can't get too close to the heat," she advises us. "You should have smelled that burnt fake hair!"

We laugh, boisterous again. Lori tells about a former member who, surviving two bone marrow transplants, is doing very well. We have two visitors, a woman named Debby who may have to get a double mastectomy and a woman named Anita who starts her first chemo treatment this Friday.

I share with Anita some of the side effects she may have, and she leans toward me, intensely interested in my experience. I hand her my business card.

"Call me if you have anymore questions or just want to talk," I suggest.

Lori makes us coffee, and I eat two sugary white cookies.

Lori, her usual outgoing self, entertains us with funny stories about the Policeman's Ball she recently attended and her job at a middle school cafeteria. We tell jokes and anticipate our new year, cancer-free.

While the others laugh, I get up and head for the bathroom. Dr. Schinke's office is empty and dark. The radiation room is also dark, its large white backlights for illuminating x-rays blending opaquely into the wall. Down the hall I see The Chemo Room—peaceful and quiet now, abandoned, waiting faithfully for tomorrow and the people who will walk through it. I can barely make out an I.V. pole standing like a sentinel beside the open door.

༺

I'll end this chapter with another breast cancer support group story, a City of Hope experience that I heard a few months after visiting Dalilah:

"White Flag of Surrender"

At the breast cancer support group tonight, Dalilah looks good. Her hair is growing back. She smiles in her shy way and tells us all that she's doing well. Marie, a heavyset woman with a short black wig, tells us about her recent bone marrow transplant experience at City of Hope.

"They gave me so much morphine for my mouth sores that I was completely out of it. One night, I took my big white panties off and hoisted them to the top of my I.V. pole. Then I walked through the halls stark naked. The nurses told me about this later; I don't remember a thing. I guess I was waving my white flag of surrender. I'm glad to be here now."

We can't help but laugh at Marie's story, and I guess we're all thinking the same thing:

we can either give in to the cancer or fight.

And so, gathered in a circle like a female version of King Arthur's Knights of the Round Table, we plan our strategies for this year's Breast Cancer Awareness Month and Walk for a Cure.

Five

Woman on a Cliff

I go through periodic episodes of paranoia (I think I have good reasons). Here is a journal entry I wrote about a year after the end of my chemo treatments:

"Phobia"

Sometimes I'm afraid to hope for good things.

I still think about accidents when I put the kids in the car. I think about kidnappings when I shop at Target. In the middle of the night, I wake up, stare at the crisscrossed ceiling, and think about radiation.

How much radiation does that computer monitor put out, anyway? Jessica sits in front of it at least a couple of hours a day. Will I open the computer room door one day to find Jessica gone, swallowed into a virtual world?

And what about the T.V. and the microwave? I can't forget those chest X-rays I had as a child...

As dawn slips through the bedroom curtains, I think about what we put in our bodies. How many hormones and other additives taint the milk and meat we eat? What kind of danger from pesticides sinks into fruit and vegetables? How can peanut butter cause cancer?

What have we created in this winding-down Twentieth Century, the great Age of Technology, that can destroy us and our children in new, clever, and unseen ways?

When Edd massages me, I hold my breath. I'm afraid to touch my body for fear I'll find another lump. When I get overheated, I worry that I'm starting those strange fevers again. I feel the inside of my mouth, where I first got a "lymphoid polyp," and wonder if that bump is a ligament or a lump. Terror grips me like a hand. All reason leaves, and I can hardly breathe as thoughts avalanche my mind:

> If I find a lump, I'll have to
> tell Edd
> get a referral to a surgeon
> wait for an appointment
> get a biopsy
> wait for the results
> conference with doctors
> endure a bone marrow transplant,
> two months in the hospital,
> and maybe die...

I dread the thought of leaving my family to stay in the hospital. I'm afraid that if I go in, I will never come out. I would get lots of rest, though. Suddenly even hungry cats with litter in their paws look like a blessing. I'll try not to complain...

I'm afraid of the morning, of having to get out of bed and face a new day. I want to stay in my nightgown, under the blankets, curled up in a fetal position, crying out to God,

Please keep me safe.

How can I get up and vacuum the house when I think at any moment our family could be torn apart?

How can anyone live with a threat like cancer hanging over her—a threat that could strike like a hidden rattlesnake?

I've got to stop lying in bed at night and thinking

What else will go wrong?

If God means to send the cancer back to me, I cannot run; I cannot hide.

Yet deep inside I feel He means to spare me.

God has protected me many times, on so many journeys

that I can't even count the number. Why should a few really difficult events make me afraid of the future?

Unable to sleep, I get up and read. The newspaper reports about killer bees spotted in Palm Springs and headed our way. I imagine the kids and I, on one of our twilight walks through country lanes, attacked by a swarm. I can see all those fuzzy, winged creatures on Jonathan's two-year-old skin and hear his screams...

Now I know I'm getting paranoid.

I understand the term phobia. What is the official name for lump-phobia and cancer-phobia?

Wait a minute. Why am I afraid of killer bees? Didn't God make bees? Couldn't He keep us safe on our walks? And if He wants us to die by killer bee stings, worry won't stop that. I'd sooner take my chances with bees than cancer, anyway.

I open my Bible and flip through the New Testament, finding the first book of John:

> "There is no fear in love;
> but perfect love casts out fear,
> because fear involves torment.
> But he who fears has not been made
> perfect in love.
>
> We love Him because He first loved us." (1 John 4:18 & 19)

If God loves me and knows what is right for me and my family, He will guide me along the best possible path. I've got to emerge from this cocoon of fear and learn to trust God's love.

༄

I also learned about fear when I was hiking with the kids in the mountains, the place where we visited and longed to make a home. Two years after my chemo treatments, I wrote:

"The Cave"

Today I take the kids hiking. We follow a trail through mossy Rainbow Creek, stepping on stones to avoid getting wet in the shallow water.

"Look, a waterfall!" Jessica, age 6, points.

Jonathan, age 3, follows her gaze briefly and then charges across the bridge.

The trail follows the side of the mountain and gradually leads downward, showing views of rocky cliffs and tree-filled valleys. I barely notice that clouds are starting to gather above us.

I wish I had brought the camera. Jessica looks cute in her new red and blue backpack, her pink hat over her long auburn ringlets. The leader of our expedition, she pauses occasionally to consult her map and check our progress.

"So we don't get lost," she tells me.

Jonathan, following her, is not much bigger than his own backpack which droops to the back of his knees. He pauses occasionally to get his squirt bottle out of his backpack and spray the trees, a bug, a rock, and the back of Jessie's neck.

We pass a rockslide area.

"Poor mountain," Jonathan says, peering over the edge at the granite boulders and tree stumps.

"Don't get too close," I warn, grabbing his hand.

"What would happen if all the trees got cut off the mountain?" Jessica wonders. "Would the mountain fall down?"

"Maybe," I explain. "Actually, the trees help hold up the dirt so that it doesn't all slide down. The trees give the animals, birds, and insects homes. Wouldn't it be sad if there were no more trees?"

"Yes," she responds, and I think of my science fiction novel, <u>Like a Tree Planted</u>.

We hike further. The clouds are thicker, and now they're turning a dark gray. We hear a distant roll of thunder. Jonathan doesn't seem bothered by the sound, but Jessica looks at me with pouty blue eyes.

"I want to go back now," she states. She has always been terrified of thunderstorms. We turn around. It's harder to walk up the trail, and I hold Jonathan's hand (despite his protests) on one side and Jessica's hand (gladly) on the other.

"Look! A Western hemlock, my favorite tree!" I exclaim, reaching out to touch the graceful, furry branches.

"I can figure out the trees for myself," Jessie says. "Please hold my hand, because I'm so scared of thunder."

We hike past the tree and underneath a cave opening that I didn't notice before. Tall and shadowy, it reminds me of a dream I had last night. I've dreamed often since I had cancer. The dreams are alike: I enter a cave where my worst fears live, etched against damp stone walls. I see lumps of cancer in people's lungs, bones, brains. I see the chemo room and the bone marrow transplant ward where people lose their hair, turn pale like ghosts, and get sores inside their mouths. I see mounds of earth in the corners—graves for the cancer patients who did not survive. I hear the sobs of children who don't understand. I smell the dusty mold of death and feel the cave's icy breathing.

My heart starts racing as blood rushes to my head.

"What's wrong, Mommy?" Jessica asks, staring.

I'm lost in the cave. Surely—somewhere—there's an opening where sunlight shines through like a beacon.

Another thunderclap sounds—closer—and I realize I've stopped in the cave's shadow and am standing in the sudden rain.

I must walk forward—past The Chemo Room, past cancer.

And then I remember. During my last chemo treatment, I wrote a Bible verse in my journal. It returns to me now:

> "The night is far spent,
> the day is at hand.
> Therefore let us cast off
> the works of darkness,
> and let us put on
> the armor of light." (Romans 13:12)

Another rumble breaks from the sky, and Jessica jumps and trembles beside me, digging her hand further in mine.

"I'm not brave, not brave at all," she laments.

"That's okay. I get scared, too," I admit, wondering if the cancer will return, if I will live to see Jessica and Jonathan grown and with children of their own. "Sometimes I feel like a lost little girl. But then I remember that I must be strong and keep hiking. We will find our way home. The Lord will protect us."

I start moving past the cave. The thunder quiets to a distant mumble, and the sky starts turning blue again. The path ahead doesn't look too rocky. It rises toward the clearing sky, bordered on each side by pine trees.

I also have Survivor's Syndrome, which I wrote about in this:

"Hitting the Van"

Kristen flies down from Washington to visit us for Spring Break. On the way home from the airport, less than a mile from the offramp to our valley home, we become involved in a freeway accident.

It's very dark (after eight). I notice a couple of cars have pulled over to the shoulder, their taillights on. I pull over and stare ahead. At this section, the freeway has two lanes for each direction, with a wide sand divider in the middle. No one has put out flares or even a flashlight, but I discern the dim outline of a van. Tilted on one side across the fast lane, its underside faces us. Before I can think what to do, I see a large white truck, which was following me, whiz past, still going about seventy miles an hour. He obviously doesn't see the van.

"Oh God, he's going to hit the van!" I cry.

The truck crashes into the van. Gray smoke rises into the night air.

"Oh God, I hope no one was in that van," I say, envisioning

a family of five, with children in carseats, meeting a fiery death.

"I've got to check," Kristen says, beside me.

We both jump out of the car, though by now Jessica and Jonathan, confused and frightened, are crying.

"Stay out of the fast lane!" I yell at Kristen's back as she rushes to put her Nursing Assistant training to use. Her long blonde hair swings to the right as she makes a sharp left turn toward the center divider.

I reach under the carseat and grab my fluorescent flashlight (Edd teases me for collecting so many flashlights). I turn on its bright light and hand it to a man named Dave who takes it and runs into the fast lane, yelling at approaching cars:

"Stop! There's been an accident!"

"What happened?" Jessica sobs.

"The white truck hit that van," I tell her. Amazingly, I feel calm, as if God's hand covers us all on this freeway.

A friendly trucker named Roger parks his semi in the slow lane so that no one can plow into my car. Another trucker parks next to him, blocking the fast lane. Their blinking amber truck lights act as flares until the flashing blue and whites of the Highway Patrol arrive.

When the fire engines park on the center divider, I set out to find Kristen (Roger watches my car). I see her near a dazed-looking Mexican who sits on the bumper of another truck, in the dirt divider. Near him I see a young man rubbing his shoulder and staring forlornly at the white truck he had been driving, which is completely smashed in front. Tools are scattered all over the asphalt.

"What happened?" I ask.

Kristen looks at me, the flashing emergency lights reflecting in her eyes. She grabs my shoulder and starts walking toward our car, explaining on the way:

"When the young guy in the white truck hit the van, it spun 360 degrees around and ended up in the slow lane, tilting over into the ditch. The guy in the white truck had only minor injuries—his shoulder strap bruised his shoulder but saved his life. He kept repeating how his boss was going to be mad about the ruined truck. After I made sure he was okay, I got him to crawl down in the ditch with me and look inside the van to see if anyone was in it because nobody seemed to know. Nobody was in it. We found out that a truck was towing the van when the trailer broke, and the van flipped on its side. After the accident, the man who was towing the van just sat on his bumper in the center divider and did nothing."

"Amazing. So nobody was seriously hurt."

"Right. The van was pouring gas all over the freeway, too."

"I'm proud of you," I say, patting Kristen's arm as we reach our car. "You must have been terrified running toward that van in the darkness, not knowing what you would find."

She gets in the car and puts her seatbelt on, and I do the same.

"I just kept thinking that I had to help whoever was in that van," she confides. "I didn't have time to feel scared."

Dave walks over and hands my flashlight back to me since the police now direct traffic. "I was on the phone when I heard the truck hit the van," he tells us. "Ten people must have used their cell phones to call 911."

I must have been the only one without a cell phone—and the only one with a flashlight.

"Thanks," I say as I take my flashlight and put it back under the seat. I start the car and move in line with others, slowly passing the accident scene.

"Welcome back to California," Kristen murmurs to herself.

As we drive past the van (still on its side), I wonder how I can stay calm in emergency situations yet freeze in terror at the thought of cancer.

Tonight I dream I'm driving alone on a dark freeway. A black van suddenly appears, blocking my lane. I slam on the brakes and stop inches away from the gleam of metal in the dark, shaking, my hands gripping the steering wheel. In the silence after screeching brakes, I begin to hear another sound, high-pitched, at regular intervals.

The sound is my own voice, screaming. I look to my left and right and see other people crash into the van.

Why did I escape? I scream through my dream, my hands still stuck to the steering wheel.

Of course, I realize that mine is an American Tragedy. I have a lot of beauty and blessing in my life, too. I didn't grow up in a country where poverty and politics prevented me from getting my next meal, obtaining health care, going to college, marrying for love, raising happy children, ice skating, going to church, buying a computer, or writing a book. I should move to Afghanistan and live with the refugees. Then I would have a better view of tragedy. But for now, I am a:

"Woman on a Cliff"

I am a woman standing on a cliff.
Wind rises from below,
from the dark and far crevasse.
Upon my face and hair it sings
blowing out my scarf like wings.

I cannot see the bottom of the cliff.
Rocks and slopes and trees
reach down in shades of gray and green.
And if they form a bridge
they stay unseen.

But I'm not frightened now
to stand here at this dizzy height.
I look up to the Summit where
the clouds half cover crystal peaks
and sunrise turns the snow to light.

I am a woman standing on a cliff.
At any time my feet could slip
and pull me fast
upon the razor tip.

But, oh, the view!
The view is worth the coldest risk.

Six

Alien

Somewhere in the midst of all my post-cancer paranoia, I decided to turn around, face the monster, stop being a victim, and fight. This happened in the year between miscarriages, when my mother-in-law died of lung cancer:

"The Alien"

One of my favorite films is a horror story. It reminds me of my fight with cancer. It's called <u>Alien</u>.

The film starts with a grim, dark, metallic setting as the camera explores a seemingly lifeless spaceship which looks like an ugly, rectangular barge. It drifts silently in space until a computer awakens its crewmembers from their frozen sleep—to answer a distress call from a nearby planet. The crew, in a shuttle, leaves the barge and lands on the planet. An exploration team puts on spacesuits and follows the distress beacon through a stormy desert and to a gigantic crashed alien vessel.

There one of the crew, Caine, finds a cargo hold filled with egg-like things beneath a glowing green sea of mist. He parts the mist and climbs down to examine one cone-like object that opens slowly like a clam. Then something like a giant crab leaps out and attaches to his helmet, shattering the face mask and sending its tentacles down his throat and into his body.

The other team members carry his still-breathing body

back to the ship. Officer-in-Charge Ripley (Sigourney Weaver) refuses to let the contaminated crewmember into the ship, but the science officer overrides her and opens the airtight door.

This is their great mistake.

Back at the mothership, the science officer and captain stretch Caine out on an exam table and discover that the alien is controlling his breathing and cannot easily be removed. They carefully slice into one of the crab-like legs that still clings to Caine's face. Alien blood drips acid through the spaceship's metal floors—through level after level—almost breaching the hull and entering space.

The alien suddenly releases Caine and dies. Caine awakens. The crew thinks all is well and enjoys a meal together. In the middle of the meal comes one of Hollywood's most famous scenes—Caine gasps and contorts his face as he grips his stomach in pain. Astounded crewmembers watch as a creature's head rips through Caine's chest, splattering blood on them and leaving Caine lifeless and twitching on the floor.

The alien's offspring scurries away and hides in the huge ship. It grows quickly, hunts down, and consumes all of the crewmembers but one. We watch through Ripley's eyes as she, left alone in the barge with the alien, tries to outsmart it and survive.

Today, as I check on my mother-in-law, I feel like Ripley inching down metallic corridors, not knowing around which bend the alien waits.

Ruth, who is 76 years old, hasn't been answering her phone.

She doesn't answer the door either. I hear the T.V., her constant companion, blast from inside the apartment. I get out my key, open the door, and peer inside. Though the sun shines outside, in here everything is dusky and stale, the curtains drawn, the windows shut.

Seeing no body stretched on the floor, I step in, holding my breath. I notice the dust and dirt that have accumulated in the corners and countertops, the pile of ashes under the sofa where she sits to watch T.V., the ash tray with its half-smoked brown cigarettes, and the black round burn marks all over the carpet. I walk silently under the stare of Ruth's handpainted artwork—a lion, a little girl, trees against mountains. Her giant horse statue regards me with unblinking eyes.

Ruth is in the bedroom, stretched out on the bed, eyes closed. Her face holds a gray pallor that shows more than old age. I hesitate a moment before trying to awaken her, wondering if she still breathes.

She takes a while to fully open her eyes. She's wearing a blue hairnet and a frayed floral nightgown. There's a cigarette burn on the front of the nightgown, above her left breast.

"Are you alright?" I ask.

"I have been sick," Ruth tells me. She raises herself on one elbow and then sits up. She grabs her trashcan and spits something into it.

"I haven't been able to pass my bowels. I haven't eaten a real meal in a month. And I've had these for two or three weeks," she says, pulling down her nightgown collar to show me a lump above her left breast. It looks like a flesh-colored golf ball sticking out of her skin. "They're all over my body."

She shows me another one in her abdomen. It is the size of a lemon and has red feeder veins going to it from all directions, nourishing it, making it grow.

"Here, feel it," she commands. She grabs my hand and puts it over the scarlet lump. It feels hard and warm to my touch.

I step back and place my hand over my mouth.

I see cancer for what it is—a crab, a dragon, an alien. It has its claws deep into Ruth, and they're sticking up from her skin for me to see.

"Why didn't you tell me how sick you were?" I ask.

She doesn't reply.

"I've got to get you to the emergency room," I decide. Ruth's light blue eyes look up at me, helpless and afraid. She knows what she's got there in her body—what those lumps mean.

As I drive Ruth to the E.R., I think of <u>Alien</u>. In its sequel, <u>Aliens</u>, Ripley is rescued from her drifting spaceship where she has been in deep sleep for fifty-seven years. She awakens to a strange world where even the daughter she left has grown old and died. She has recurring nightmares of the alien hiding inside her, feeding on her, killing her as it emerges. She wakes up each night, drenched with sweat and clutching her chest.

Ripley discovers that The Company has sent families to colonize the alien's breeding planet, perhaps not knowing what lay dormant there. The colonists have not been heard from lately. The Company realizes that they must have discovered the alien ship with its deadly cargo of eggs. They decide to send in the marines. Sick of trying to hide from the terror, Ripley decides to join the marines. She goes on the offensive. She becomes the hunter.

The marines face a whole hive of aliens and soon find out what they're up against. The aliens are like the essence of evil: relentless, merciless, tireless. They have one desire: kill the humans. After all of Ripley's marine friends have been killed or wounded, Ripley decides to rescue a little girl named Newt. Ripley arms herself with a cannon rifle, bullets, grenades, and a flamethrower. Alone, Ripley enters caves where aliens, in insect-like stages of development, feed on human hosts. She breaches the inner chamber full of alien eggs. She sets the chamber ablaze and, like a desperate mother, faces the alien queen in a life-or-death duel.

Near the film's end, Ripley—exhausted and bleeding and covered with sweat—holds Newt on the edge of a metal scaffold. Explosions and debris surround them. The alien queen, furious that Ripley destroyed her eggs, advances with her horned head and pinchers waving. Ripley tells Newt, "Close your eyes, baby." Then the rescue ship appears behind them, hovering amid the flames. Its robot pilot lowers the stairs, and Ripley and Newt climb to safety seconds before the planet's surface explodes in a nuclear cloud.

That's how I feel when I think about surviving cancer.

Seven

Question Mark

On February 11, 1997, seven months after the end of chemotherapy, I wrote this in my journal:

"Glad to Be Alive"

I take the kids outside, so they can work off some energy.

It's a lovely afternoon, cool, sunny, with an edge of white clouds along the horizon. I follow Jessica under the eucalyptus tree at the back gate—the tree with branches that hang down like hair. Jessie grabs a handful of branches and shows me how she can swing all by herself, forward and back among the slender leaves. Jonathan follows us into the tree's interior and picks up pink flowers like tiny brushes. It's almost spring.

We leave the tree's shelter and wander the fenceline, peering over at the neighbor's goats and dogs. The kids turn and run across the field which is lushly green with new weeds. Jessica wears her pink sweatshirt, spattered with mud, and her blue snowboots that she got for Christmas. Jonathan wears Jessie's old evergreen sweatshirt and pink rainboots. His diapers sag a little between his legs as he jogs across the uneven ground.

I want to go in the house and sleep but instead take the kids for a walk. I strap a protesting Jonathan into his big-wheeled, go-anywhere stroller. Jessie, tired already from our yard ramblings, sits on the metal basket frame in back of

Jonathan. She holds on to the yellow bar above her. We head for neighbor Ray's hill that is bordered by eucalyptus trees.

"My hands are cold, Mommy," she says. The sun has dipped past the hills, and we see a crescent moon shining against the dark blue sky.

"Moon, moon!" Jonathan declares, pointing.

I place my hands over Jessica's, warming them. I'm wearing my wine-colored corduroy dress with a denim vest and my Canadian snowboots, so I'm not cold.

"Did you know that you are a gift from God?" I ask Jessica who stares up at me. "Before you were born, I stood at the window and saw you in the moon."

"You saw me in the moon?" she asks.

"Yes. And the moonlight filtered down through the blinds and onto my face, and I knew you would come and live with us."

Jessica turns and looks at the moon again. I push further up the hill.

Jonathan leans forward toward the stroller wheels and shows me layer upon layer of curls in the back of his head. He'll be twenty months tomorrow.

"I want bottle, please," he says, turning to look at me.

"Let's go for a walk," I reply. "Look, horsie!"

Ray's chocolate-colored Shetland pony seems indifferent to us. She stands at the top of the field, looking moonward.

"I want pookie, please," Jonathan tries a new request.

"I'll give you a cookie when we get home. Look, doggie!"

Distracted from food and drink, Jonathan leans toward the neighbor's golden lab puppy who jumps up and kisses him.

"I want doggie, please," Jonathan says.

I walk past the puppy, feeling the wind against my face and the sweat of real exercise as I push the heavy load upward against new mud and wet grass. We follow the line of Ray's eucalyptus trees. Light fades quickly from the sky now, and the moon shines through the tree branches, seeming to move with us as we stare upward.

How the sky glows in twilight, I realize, as I glance from

the moon to my two children. At the hilltop, I stop the stroller and walk forward. Bending over Jonathan, I brush his cheek and sing,

"Jesus loves me."

"Jesus loves me," Jonathan repeats, and Jessica adds the verses Jonathan cannot say. The last evening light illumines our faces as she sings. And I think,

I'm glad to be alive.

❧

A few days later I discovered I was pregnant with my first miscarriage.

Sometimes my life feels like one big question mark.

Have you ever stood on top of a mountain and heard the wind blow in the trees above you? When it sweeps down to your face, it feels as though the very stars have sent it—like a kiss blown earthward. Have you ever looked through that high, clear atmosphere (where even gravity is slightly less) and stared at the Big Dipper, northward, shaped like a giant question mark?

I had five miscarriages in four years, after my chemotherapy treatments. Three were early (at about 6 weeks)—just a lot of bleeding and emotions. One was at almost 3 months, and I had a D & C in the hospital. My friend, Dr. Ann, prayed with me before I went under the anesthesia. When I woke up from surgery, I was sobbing—deep heaves from the center of my being. A nurse patted my hand and said soothing words I do not remember.

The worst miscarriage was in December of 1997, when I lost baby Michael at four months. He was born at home, in the middle of the night. My water broke. I thought I had peed the bed and ran to the bathroom. Baby Michael slipped out with no pain. He looked perfectly formed, though very still and pale— small enough to hold in the palm of my hand. His little arm was pinned behind his back as he floated in the Tupperware dish where I put him. His face looked like Jonathan's—smooth and angelic, impish and beautiful, but the eyes forever unseeing.

We lived in the valley then. Edd buried Michael in the yard under a silk tree that silhouetted the distant mountains.

Two nights later, I ended up in the E. R., hemorrhaging. But the huge placenta passed, and I didn't need a D & C.

All five miscarriages were heartbreaking and miserable—whether they happened shortly after I told everyone the news or months later.

Instead of having miscarriages, I should have just peacefully headed into menopause. I shouldn't have believed Dr. Schinke when he said that I probably could have another child. There weren't enough clinical studies to prove that...

But I never felt or looked old. I was still having regular periods and all the normal hormonal things for a woman of child-bearing age. I often saw women who looked older than me, their faces well lined and their bellies visibly pregnant. And I thought to myself, I bet I'm in better shape than she is. I can ice skate! I can get out on that rink with my children and skate for hours, forward and backward, doing my edges and spins.

A fertility doctor even told me that I had a "good egg reserve" despite my age and the chemo. Too bad he didn't know those eggs were damaged. I guess it's not how young you look on the outside that counts.

After my five miscarriages, I buried my feelings deep. I wanted to be numb. I wanted to sleep. But I couldn't stop the <u>dreams</u>.

I avoided pregnant women and babies. I didn't talk about anything to do with conception or childbirth. What was the point of stirring up painful feelings? Would talking bring even one of those lost babies back? I knew that no power on earth could do that. And God wasn't likely to, either.

At other times, the voice of practical realism would come to me: what's the big deal? Lots of women have miscarriages. Lots of women pay to have abortions. It's just a bunch of blood and premature cells, anyway. Get over it.

Sometimes I wanted to take that casual view, but I couldn't. I was raised Catholic, though since I was a teenager, I've mainly been going to Protestant churches. I have a personal relationship with Christ—who brought me like a newborn baby into His kingdom. I can't help but believe, as Psalm 139 indicates, that life begins when an egg is fertilized by the sperm. After all, it starts to grow immediately. It has its own DNA. It splits from one cell into many, attaching to the lining of the uterus, starting to form limbs, beating its tiny heart that shows up on a sonogram like a pulsing star.

But if it's so alive, so something other than my own body, why does it die before it has a chance to be born?

> I go back to Psalm 139, a psalm of David:
> "For You formed my inward parts;
> You covered me
> in my mother's womb.
>
> I will praise You,
> for I am fearfully and wonderfully made;
> marvelous are Your works,
> and that my soul knows very well.
>
> My frame was not hidden from You,
> when I was made in secret,
> and skillfully wrought
> in the lower parts of the earth.
>
> Your eyes saw my substance,
> being yet unformed.
> And in Your book
> they all were written,
> the days fashioned for me,
> when as yet there were none of them!"

Did all my miscarriages serve no purpose on this earth? Were the books of their life all blank pages?

Why, if God can do anything, did He bring so many miscarriages into my life? Couldn't he have saved one, just one of those five lost babies?

The fifth one seemed too much. Each miscarriage seemed connected somehow to all the suffering in my life, from childhood on—even to all the suffering of all the people on earth. And so the fifth one seemed multiplied beyond measure.

How can the miracle of love and conception—of the basic beginnings of life—go wrong? How can the womb become a tomb?

Sometimes I feel like my five miscarriages were a big joke. If so, am I the punchline? Or the punching <u>bag</u>?

Why does God let us suffer?

Many people have asked that question. The book of Job is one of the oldest books in the Old Testament. I always identified with Job. He had everything: big houses, land, flocks, respect, health, children. In one day, he lost it all. Even his wife told him, as he sat in a pile of ashes and used a piece of pottery to scrape the painful, oozing boils all over his skin,

"Curse God and die."

Job replied,

"The Lord gives, and the Lord takes away. Blessed is the name of the Lord."

Still, Job asked God questions.

David asked questions, too. God promised that he would be king of Israel, but David spent years hiding out in wilderness caves, running from King Saul who hunted him like a dog. Read the Psalms. You'll find some of David's complaining and questioning.

Rabbi Harold S. Kushner wrote a book called <u>When Bad Things Happen to Good People</u>. One of his points is that it's nothing personal, just life, just the way things are. If you're in the way when a car speeds toward you, you'll get hurt. Physics. Cause and effect. God isn't personally out to hurt you.

But I believe in a personal God who is involved in my life, who is all-powerful and all-knowing. Therefore, I come to the conclusion that He let those five miscarriages happen to me.

But why? So I can write a book and touch people's lives and have some of them tell me,

"You're such an inspiration."

A cold keyboard and a few compliments seem like poor consolation.

You can see why my life is a question mark.

Eight

Kauai and New York

2001 was a tough year for us. We had trouble with my brother-in-law and the house he was renting from us in the valley where we used to live before moving to the mountains. We had to move him and his family out so that we could sell the place. We had to clean up after him. We spent Easter vacation scrubbing places a person wouldn't want to look at.

Then came the long summer. Edd stressed out over his job, the commute down the mountain, and the possibility of buying a bigger house (with a garage and an actual yard instead of just a slope). I had searing headaches and a root canal. I was continuing to do homeschool, write when I could, and go to the ice skating rink several times a week. We were involved with our church but maybe a little burned out. I wasn't making any money at writing, and the bills (thanks in a large part to Edd's brother) were piling up.

So we did the logical thing. We took a vacation in Hawaii at the end of summer. We spent two wonderful, relaxing weeks in Kauai. Here's what I wrote about it:

"Bouncing Back"

My life has always been a series of bouncing back and forth between one place and another. Florida, Maine, London, Los Angeles...

One college professor said I would make a good cultural anthropologist because I fit in everywhere I go, and I know how to follow a map. It's true. I take a new place, new culture, and new language on me like a chameleon changes with the color of her tree.

But it has become harder to bounce from place to place, especially when the speed of an airplane takes me across time zones.

Last week I was in Kauai. We drove as far as we could from one end of the Garden Isle to another, to where the Na Pali Coast cut off the road—with its sheer green cliffs cut like cathedral spires above the sea. We drove to Weimea Canyon, "The Grand Canyon of the Pacific," where Edd posed on the brink with the kids so that I could take a photo . . . My old paranoia returned. As I snapped the shutter, I could feel the force of gravity pulling at my children. I imagined Jonathan slipping and tumbling 3000 feet down the orange rocks, so I grabbed him by the hand and retreated to the rental car.

We drove to Kokee Park, in the mountains above Weimea at 4,000 feet, where someone planted fur trees a hundred years ago. The white cool mist contrasted with the gold sand beach far below—Poli Hale, "House of Fire," where the air is so hot and dry you can barely breathe, you get a sunburn in ten minutes, and the dark blue water breaks against the cliffs.

At the end of Kokee, Jessica and I hiked on a muddy trail along the Na Pali ridge. We saw tree ferns as tall as we were, admiring their centers curled up like springs we could unwind to touch the spores. We pulled ourselves up by tree roots to Pihea Vista. From there we could see, between the cathedral peaks to the west, green valleys once covered by lost Hawaiian villages. To the east, we could see swampland jungle—a mass of short grayish trees with no path downward. Above that, its summit always covered by clouds, rose Mount Waialele, where the first Hawaiians fled to escape their Polynesian invaders.

Mount Waialele is the wettest spot on earth. It is the source of a hundred waterfalls that rush thousands of feet down its crater sides, each leading to a river that journeys across the island to the sea. Edd took the kids fishing so that I could ride a helicopter into Waialele. The pilot hovered inside the crater, near the "Weeping Wall" where water constantly cascades down in one continuous sheet against the rock.

Edd, the children, and I walked on beaches where the sand was clean and the water clear, where no smog lingered on the horizon and no skyscrapers rose in the distance. The children played at the spot where a river joined the ocean, mixing its fresh water with salty surf. We drove past Kilauea Lighthouse, Princeville, and Hanalei Bay—to the end of the road on the northwest side of the island. We walked into caves cut into cliffrock thousands of years ago by a higher tide. Millions of tons of rock stretched above our heads as the vast end of the cave disappeared in water and tunnels.

We found Ke'e, a bay with sand on one side and a coral reef on the other. We went snorkeling, Jonathan so excited at his new world that he swam ahead of me, chasing rainbow-colored fish. I had to grab his hand and pull him back against the current, stroking hard with my long fins. Jessica, wide-eyed at the mass of rock and waving anemones and silver fish the size of her arm, yanked at me and stood up to scream,

"Be careful! Watch out for the waves!"

She could see the rocky point where the wild Na Pali touched the surf.

We returned to the North Shore, to craft shops and dress shops and outside cafes where the locals hung out and exchanged surfing stories. Edd learned the sign for "hang loose," his pinky finger and thumb stretched out almost like a hitch-hiker's, a reminder to relax and enjoy the Hawaiian life, the spirit of Aloha, of nobody cares what you look like, of relax and wear your swimsuit to the grocery store.

We watched dancers do the Hula, stories told like sign language through body moves and hand motions.

We learned Hawaiian words, how to pronounce all those vowels one at a time. We learned to walk outside in the rain, with no umbrella, and to slide our feet across the wet grass, among the tropical flowers that look like birds painted orange and black and yellow and green. We had lunch with peacocks, and the male spread his feathers for us and danced.

Edd and I became closer, renewing our relationship as God renews the land with rain. We had time to relax together without having to clean house, teach, answer the phone, or rush off to appointments. At night, trade winds blew across the island, swaying palm trees outside our bedroom window and wafting in the scent of plumeria flowers.

Kauai felt so much like home to us that we looked at real estate and bought another timeshare.

I admit that it was humid and hot, mosquitoes bit us constantly, and the prices were not cheap. It's hard for the locals to make a living on the island. The youth don't have enough to do at night when they can't surf. People tend to abandon their rusty cars on the sides of roads. But we loved Kauai anyway. Who wouldn't?

After we flew away from Kauai, we spent a whirlwind weekend in Maui while I attended the very expensive and elitist Maui Writers' Conference. Then we flew back to California—in a big jet full of passengers. Then we got the post-vacation blues as more bills piled up, our dusty house needed cleaning, the laundry looked like a mountain, the empty refrigerator needed refilling, a new college semester began, and I still wasn't making money selling books.

A week after we returned from Hawaii, on September 11, terrorists attacked New York. We watched in horror—along with everyone else in the country—as two airliners smashed into the twin towers of the World Trade Center:

"A Good World"

On September 11, when I first heard the news about America being attacked by terrorists, I couldn't turn the T.V. off. I just had to know what happened. I tried to shield my children by sending them to their room. But they had already caught glimpses of airplanes slamming into skyscrapers, and they snuck back to the living room to watch. They wanted to be with me, so I let them stay.

Jonathan, age 6, started playing loudly with his toy cars as if to drown out the news. Jessica, almost 9, sprawled on the sofa, her eyes steady on the T.V. screen. She moaned,

"We just flew in an airplane like that. Why do I have to know about this? Why isn't it a good world?"

I tried to assure her that the world still has lots of good in it. Didn't we just get back from Hawaii, where we snorkeled with the rainbow fish above a coral reef? Don't we live in a small town on top of a mountain where we're safe?

"And didn't God protect us last Valentine's Day when the roof on the ice rink collapsed?" I reminded her. "We had a homeschool party planned for that day, but the rink was closed because there was so much snow in the parking lot, and both snowplows were broken. God watched over all the little ice skaters."

"Why didn't God protect New York?" she asked.

I didn't know what to say. We had heard of one hijacked plane that didn't hit its target. How many others were there? Will we ever know who was protected?

"Maybe you could help those people who were hurt—by praying for them and sending some of your money to the Red Cross," I suggested, trying to be practical.

She stared silently at me, her blue eyes wide behind her pink-rimmed glasses. A show came on where counselors offered to speak with upset people. Jessica tried calling, but the lines were busy.

"Well, whatever evil we have brought into this world, whatever suffering God allows, He will make right someday. Like we studied in the Book of Revelation, there will be a new heaven and a new earth where no pain or death exists—where everything is more beautiful than we can imagine."

This helped a little, but heaven seemed an abstract future to my little girl as she saw the present reality. I finally turned the T.V. off and read something simple that she could understand—Psalm 23. She calmed down, the words seeping into her mind—images of Jesus, the Shepherd, guarding His flock. She relaxed and waited for Dad to come home from work. He was always better at reassuring her than I was. And he did, gathering her up in his big embrace. Jonathan had already fallen asleep on the sofa, and we tucked both children safely in their brightly colored beds.

I went to bed feeling sick to my stomach for all those people in New York. I used to go to school there, hanging out in Manhattan where my uncle's family lived. I used to stand on top of the Empire State Building, look at the Twin Towers, and wonder:

"in an emergency, how could people get down all those flights of stairs?"

Late that night, I dreamed of being in one of those hijacked airplanes. It flew down the Hudson River, banked over the Statue of Liberty, and headed toward the World Trade Center. I felt the horrible sudden realization before the airplane hit the building, swallowed up by metal and glass in a blaze of 2000-degree fire. Then I stood on the ground, looking up at falling debris as people ran for cover: secretaries, stock brokers, waitresses, bankers—and the police and firefighters who came rushing to their aid.

These are our workers. They woke up early to do their job, never knowing the evil that men were about to unleash into their good world.

Then I wandered through empty, shelled-out buildings, searching for survivors—for a familiar, living face like my cousin Larry Petrillo whose friend worked at the World Trade Center.

When I awoke, I glanced at the alarm clock's red numbers and asked:

"Why do I need to know about this? Why isn't it a good world?"

I drifted back to sleep and found myself at our ruined ice rink. I stood at the edge, staring at tons of snow and metal covering the once-smooth surface. I remembered how it used to be—a high, graceful roof arcing upward with no walls, the open forest, sunlight slanting down onto the ice, mist rising slightly from the cold, and the smell of pine trees and snow. The little skaters would wear red wool caps or glittering blue dresses, their blades cutting into the ice like whispers, the wind brushing their faces like wings. They would spin or jump into the air, free from the earth for a second before landing and skating away.

Then I saw the Twin Towers falling, and Jesus standing tall above them—the Shepherd welcoming souls into his widespread arms.

And He spoke to the workers:

"Come to Me, all who are weary and heavy laden, and I will give you rest."

༄

A few weeks after September 11, I found out, unbelievably, that I was pregnant. What a time to get pregnant—with America recovering from terrorists attacks and going to war. Edd and I hopefully imagined a strong boy to be born in June—a boy who would serve God in a special way.

So when I had my fifth miscarriage the end of October, it just didn't feel right. Not that the other four felt right. But this baby seemed meant to be: life out of destruction, hope out of despair.

We were both, no doubt, thinking of baby Michael who died at four months prenatal and whom we buried in our valley yard.

When I got my CAT-scan shortly after I discovered I had cancer, the x-ray technician called me over after the ordeal and showed me the glowing monitor. There, in white against black, was the perfect circle of a follicle in my ovary.

"You'll ovulate from your left side soon," she stated.

Why did she show me? I wondered. Next week I start chemotherapy, and that egg will be fried by the chemicals. Oh, God, couldn't you protect one last egg—give us one more baby someday? I silently prayed as she turned off the monitor.

Six months after chemotherapy ended, I took a nap one

afternoon and dreamed that an angel, like a bright light, came to me and asked,

Will you have another child?

Jonathan was only one and a half. I wasn't longing for another baby. I was still recovering from the whole cancer ordeal. I could think of a thousand good, logical reasons why I should not get pregnant again.

Yes, my heart replied to the question.

After five years and five miscarriages, I think I must have seriously misunderstood that dream. Or maybe there's another meaning to it.

That October, I had to face the finality of my fifth miscarriage. My body, which had felt so full of life the week before, had emptied itself. I went to church the week after my miscarriage, and people kept giving me hugs and trying to encourage me.

"How do you feel?" people asked.

"OK physically. I went ice skating yesterday. I bounce back pretty well," I replied.

But I really didn't want to talk about it.

I wondered how everyone knew about my latest miscarriage. I had told only a couple of friends. Then someone pointed out that it was announced in the church bulletin—as a prayer request.

Well, I had told everyone at church that I was pregnant, so they had the right to know that I was not. But there in the church bulletin in black letters—so final and obvious!

My life is an open book.

With all those hugs at church, I kept up a brave front. But when Nina hugged me, I burst into sobs.

Nina is my friend from Russia. She has lived in America for only four years. She has short red hair, a thin figure, and likes to wear trendy clothes. We met at Wednesday morning Community Bible Study—almost two years ago, after my fourth miscarriage. She has a daughter Jessie's age and a two-year-old. She found out she was pregnant again the same time I did. We were both going to have a June baby. Then she found out she was carrying twins. When she heard about my miscarriage, she found me in the church gym on a Wednesday night and gave me a big hug.

"Maybe you can adopt Russian baby," she suggested. "My sister lives there, and I know attorney. Maybe I can help."

Between my sobs, I thanked her for the idea. Perhaps Edd and I will go all the way to Russia to find a baby. But somehow that just doesn't feel right...

I think that God's grace is a messy business. He sends His grace to the darkest places, the bloodiest battles, the weakest moans. One of my favorite stories in the Bible is the one about the prostitute who came into the Jewish leader's house where Jesus was a dinner guest. Somehow she got past the gatekeepers and arrived where Jesus sat. There she knelt, weeping. Her face must have been caked with makeup, white powder against black eyeliner and rouge cheeks. Her gold jewelry reflected the lamplight as she bent to wash the dusty feet of Jesus with her tears. She loosened her long hair from its clasp and used it to wipe the mud off His feet. She kissed his feet. Then she broke an alabaster jar of expensive perfume and poured it over Him, anointing Him beforehand for his burial (see Luke chapter 7).

The dinner host had not shown Jesus good hospitality that day. He didn't give Jesus water to wash with or kiss Him or anoint Him with oil. But the sinful woman did, and Jesus forgave her sins. He even added:

> "Wherever this gospel is preached
> throughout the whole world,
> what this woman did
> will also be spoken of
> as a memorial to her." (Mark 14:9)

My friend Cherie knows about God's messy grace. She has four children—three girls and a boy. They are best friends with my own children. Cherie and her husband Bill wanted another boy. She gave birth to a dead one six weeks before his due date. Her story is one of the worst cases. She carried that child for seven and a half months. When he suddenly ceased moving inside her, she found out his heart had stopped. She went into labor. When he was born still and lifeless, her scream echoed through our mountain hospital.

God was there in that hospital room with Cherie and Bill, somehow giving hope of life beyond death.

God's grace also reached into the horrible wreckage of New York. People from all over the country came to help or sent gifts. Rescue workers and cleanup crews labored through the long days and nights.

For a week after September 11, airports across the country were closed. It was eerie to stand on our mountaintop and see no jetliners pass overhead, silver and graceful against the dark blue sky as they headed across the continent. The sky was quiet, as if in mourning.

Now, despite the possible hazards of flying, I want to take the first plane back to Kauai. I want to stand on the cliff at Kilauea, with the view of curving coastline on both sides and the waves crashing against white rock. I want to stand by that lighthouse at the northernmost point in the Hawaiian islands, the mountains and waterfalls and mist behind me, and watch the waves roll in. I want to feel the trade wind on my face, wiping away my tears, bathing me in forgetfulness.

Instead, in my mind and my dreams, I keep going back to New York—to the pile of rubble that was the World Trade Center. Nearly two months later, it still smolders as the smoke from tons of glass and metal and paper—and three thousand lives—rises into the air. I want to journey, like a pilgrim, to that spot. I want to place a flower there—my memorial for my fifth miscarriage, for yet another life gone from the earth.

Nine

Where Do the Unborn Go?

When I had my first miscarriage, it was less than a year since I finished chemotherapy. That pregnancy lasted about six weeks. Since the chemicals were still fresh in my body, I figured the fetus had no chance. Still, I grieved—perhaps as much for the fact that I had endured cancer as for the fact I lost a child. Jonathan wasn't even two years old yet, and he would sit in my lap and comfort me when I cried, his bottle dangling out of his mouth and his curls tickling my chin.

This is what I wrote after my first miscarriage:

"Where Do the Unborn Go?"

I think of my mother. She is dead now, but I remember what she looked like when she was my age. She accented her blonde curls with colored scarves and wore fashionable clothes like a movie star. Her blue eyes were piercing bright, and she painted her lips pink.

She miscarried when I was thirteen, while she was married to the stepfather I hated.

"A little lump of tissue just plopped into the toilet," she told me a few days later. "It looked like a jellyfish, almost alive in the water. I caught it in a glass jar filled with water. I didn't want it to dry out. We're creatures of the sea, Lonna. I wish the baby had lived. I'll never have another."

Perhaps she saw ahead, to those years when my brother and I would be gone, her new husband would be dead like my father, and she would long for a living child.

I remember my mother's tears when she spoke of the miscarriage, salt water like the unborn child's home. She could have flushed the fetus down the toilet, out of sight, unburied, unremembered. But I think she did the right thing to save the unborn, admire its tissue like translucent filaments, like tentacles reaching through an ocean, grasping toward sunlight dotted by plankton, dusty, murky, bright—the sea in a world never touched, never known.

Where do the Unborn go? I wondered when my mother told me her story. Where do the Unborn go? I wonder now. Their terrestrial bodies go down the drain, into the earth, or into a vial where slowly their tissue dissolves until all you see is a tube of water behind glass, unspotted and clear and cold.

※

But there must be more than that. I flip through my old journals to something I wrote nine years ago when I was pregnant with my daughter Jessica:

"Little Lives and Deaths"

She tries to pull ahead of me into the parking space—driving fast in her yellow Volkswagen, her boyfriend beside her. I'm not about to give up the space, since neither the Chevy pickup nor me is very maneuverable. Eight months pregnant, big as a house, I lumber out of the truck behind the young couple heading for Dr. Wong's office.

They take their place across from me in the waiting room. She can't be more than sixteen—skinny, red-haired, freckled. She wears a "beach bum" t-shirt, frayed shorts, sandals. Her dark-haired boyfriend, also thin and not much taller than she, doesn't look up from his magazine. She glances at me sideways: me, the very pregnant woman, at least twice her size and age.

My obnoxious belly, in its purple maternity top, resembles an overgrown grape.

She fills out the forms and hands the receptionist the necessary cash (all new twenty-dollar bills). Then she waits, showing her boyfriend magazine pictures.

I watch from behind my notebook, wonder if these two knew what life doors they opened when they had sex. I can't imagine them as parents. How could I block their way to this plum-colored office with its Chinese vases, Mozart music, and walls hung with photos of babies Dr. Wong delivered? How could I beg her to keep her child? Her own wrists are narrow as a baby's thigh. Her hazel eyes flutter behind glossy magazine pictures. She sees high-fashion models with perfect mascara and long red nails.

The nurse takes the girl in, alone. My turn follows shortly, and after the usual blood pressure, urine sample, and weight check (well, she's a big baby), I wait in the corner room, which is peach-colored. I sit demurely on the exam table, wondering when our baby will "drop," wondering what questions to ask Dr. Wong. Just four more weeks! I wait, write a little, fetch a drink of water, visit the bathroom again, wait. I examine the waiting room cupboards and drawers, find the usual medical stuff (long Q-tips, gauze, syringes, plastic gloves...). Over an hour later I wander to the reception desk. Nurse Maria tells me Dr. Wong just had an "emergency" involving a "routine procedure."

I glance at the "special" room and guess that the redhead bled or went into shock. I see Dr. Wong emerge, smiling apologetically. He assures me he'll be with me in a moment as he walks down the hallway. He leaves the door ajar. I spy the girl's white feet stretched at the end of the exam table. The nurse says the boyfriend can come in now.

I wonder what Dr. Wong did with the fetal tissue and the girl's blood. I watch him down the hall as he scribbles notes on a chart. He looks so clean and professional in his white smock and glasses. He works miracles, opening women's blocked tubes with lasers to help women conceive, developing sonogram pictures, delivering babies. He performs abortions too. How strange to deal with little lives and deaths all day.

He is our servant. We pay him highly. He does only what we ask.

Back in the peach exam room, Dr. Wong cuts the visit short, listening to my baby's "strong" heartbeat, measuring her, telling me again she'll weigh nine pounds. He says she hasn't fully dropped yet. He says she'll probably be on time, though I can't imagine getting any bigger.

Well, she's happy in there—flourishing, kicking so hard my belly quakes with inside footprints. She's in no hurry to emerge. I won't rush her.

And the redhaired teenager? The nurse must be helping her sit up, handing her a glass of orange juice, telling her what bleeding to expect. The nurse will probably recommend rest and dispense antibiotics. The boyfriend will drive the girl home.

I leave the office before the girl emerges from the special room, climb into the pickup, and drive down the freeway. The baby kicks me as wind blows through open windows. Sunlight on my dirty windshield spatters the view ahead.

After my second miscarriage, I had a nightmare about the Unborn:

"The Haunted Nursery"

I doze a little and find myself in the yard of a huge Victorian house. It glows from within through stained glass windows. I crunch through snow toward the carved wood banisters of a porch, up the stairs, and to a tall door. Turning the brass doorknob, I enter and look up at a chandelier. Crystal prisms reflect colors on the white-walled entryway. A parquet wood floor leads to a wide living room laden with plush white carpet, heavy drapes, and glass cabinets full of curious silver objects.

A curving staircase descends toward me. Light shines

down from the floor above, and I hear a baby's cry. As I climb the carpeted stairs, the cry grows louder, more insistent.

"I'm coming," I call to the disconsolate child.

At the balcony I turn left down a hallway, drawn by the cry. I pass several rooms with open doorways that display postered beds covered by quilts, nightstands with lamps and doilies, and windows covered by lacy curtains.

My feet keep following the cushioned carpet, bouncing almost, as I walk down the long hall to the last room on the left. The door opens as I approach, and the crying seems to push against my chest as I enter.

It is a nursery, the most beautiful I have ever seen. Antique furniture, stacked neatly with toys and clothes, lines the room beneath watercolor paintings of mothers cradling their babies. I see no windows. In the center of the room stands a bassinet, a large round one covered with gauzy white material. Sheer white silk domes the bassinet, with a drooping satin bow on top.

I reach out my hand to part the material and see the crying baby within. An aborted fetus of about fifteen weeks, all bloody and cut up, lies on a mattress.

"I didn't abort you," I say, fascinated and repelled by the sight but unafraid.

"Your sisters did," the thin voice replies.

"Then why do you haunt *me*?" I ask.

The only answer is a plaintive wail that echoes through the house. The haunted nursery begins to collapse like strands of tissue paper around me. I awake.

Where do the Unborn go? I read about Christ's resurrection power, from 1 Corinthians 15:

"There are celestial bodies and
terrestrial bodies:
but the glory of the celestial is one,
and the glory of the terrestrial is another...

So also is the resurrection of the dead.
The body is sown in corruption;
it is raised in power...

So when this corruptible
has put on incorruptible,
and this mortal
has put on immortality,
then shall be brought to pass
the saying that is written:
'Death is swallowed up
in victory.'"

I think all the little cast-off creatures—the miscarriages and abortions—have a celestial body now. They wait for us, untouched by the corruptions of this earth.

Ten

Inspiration

Sometimes people ask me where I get inspiration. One of the places is Hollywood. Don't get me wrong; I know there's a lot of bad stuff coming out of Hollywood. But there are also certain films, or scenes from films, that are like art and literature—beautiful and wise.

From <u>The Sound of Music</u> I learned that "when God closes a door, He always opens a window." I also identify with Maria as she wanders around the mountainsides with a bunch of children following her.

From <u>Ladyhawk</u> I learned that, though a situation seems hopeless; though you come within inches of touching your heart's desire as the sun rises over the mountains (only to see your hawk fly away), God can break the curse at last.

From the <u>Alien</u> movies, I learned how to describe what fighting cancer is like. From <u>Galaxy Quest</u>, I learned "never give up; never surrender."

After baby Michael died just before Christmas four years ago, I was (to say the least) depressed. I ate spice cookies, drank Earl Grey tea, wandered around the house in my robe, and sat by the fireplace for hours. During that time I learned my greatest lesson ever from a movie:

"The Robe"

Tonight, tired and depressed, I sit in front of the fireplace and watch the beautiful blazing fire Edd made.

Edd's reading a literature book at the kitchen table, preparing for the spring semester at college. I feel like pouting alone for awhile (Edd will notice my mood eventually, set me on the sofa next to him, and massage my feet).

Flame spits up from the logs, crackling into sparks that ascend the chimney and fly out into the night sky. I watch the yellow/orange/red/blue colors of fire as it dances in front of me.

Everything dies, I chant to myself as the flame crackles and the charred logs collapse into ashes.

How did Martha feel when her brother Lazarus died? She had sent a message to Jesus to come, but He was busy preaching and healing the sick and did not arrive until Lazarus had been dead for four days. When she heard Jesus was near, she went to meet him on the road.

"Lord, if You had been here, my brother would not have died," she said.

Jesus replied,

"I am the resurrection and the life.
He who believes in Me,
though he may die, he shall live.
And whoever lives and believes in Me
shall never die. Do you believe this?

She answered, "Yes, Lord, I believe that You are the Christ, the Son of God, who is to come into the world."

Martha's sister Mary also came to meet Jesus, along with a crowd of mourners. When Jesus saw them weeping, He also wept. Then He went to Lazarus' tomb, had the people roll away the stone, and called,

"Lazarus, come forth!"

The dead man came out, bound hand and foot with gravecloths. Jesus told the people,

"Loose him, and let him go." (from John 11)

All things die, but Christ can make them rise again.

As I gaze into the flames, Jessica runs around the house on all fours, her butt up in the air, meowing like a cat.

"What does the cow say?" she stops to ask me, reaching for her cow doll in its gingham dress.

"She says 'Can I sleep with you tonight, Jessica?'"

"I'm tired of always sleeping with her. Why does she want to sleep with me all the time?"

"Because you're her mother."

"No, I'm not. I just take care of her," she insists.

"Well, she thinks you're her mother."

"Oh," she says and goes into the dining room to sit beside Edd and read her Dr. Seuss books.

I enjoy my new vocation as Cow Interpreter.

Jonathan runs through the house with his bottom bare, carrying the green potty bowl full of pee-pee to "show daddy."

He's still my Consolation, my baby, whose small hands grasp mine through his crib slats at night. When I change him, I lean over his little body and tickle him. He squeals as I poke his neck. His shoulders fit into the cup of my hand. I wonder, in years to come, what other feminine hands will caress him.

He's a sweet brat, sticking his tongue out at me and saying "no" when I tell him to put the potty bowl back. Then he smiles in an attempt to disarm my wrath.

"I want my buggies!" he demands. I set him in his "spot" (the green chair) and fetch the plastic jar full of plastic bugs. He watches the flames with me for awhile and falls asleep. I sit back down in front of the fireplace and remember other things Jonathan says to me.

"I hate that movie," he'll state when we watch the black and white version of Jane Austin's <u>Pride and Prejudice</u>.

"But I <u>like</u> food," he'll protest when I try to take away my picture-filled cookbook that he pulled down from a shelf.

"Where's Jesus?" he'll ask, getting up to stand at the wooden childgate and look outside through the screen door.

I think about things I bought for baby Michael who died four months into the womb: a washer and dryer, a headset cordless telephone, a pewter baby cup, and a little white bib with poinsettia flowers and letters that spell "baby's first Christmas."

Hot tears start to wander annoyingly down my cheeks. My nose gets stuffy again, and I blow it repeatedly. My head begins to ache. I hate crying.

I try reasoning with God about why he should give us another baby. I could continue to annoy Dr. Ing with calls in the middle of the night. I could still attend MOPS (Mothers of Preschoolers) meetings. I could help populate the church nursery.

Jessica prays for a baby. If you don't answer my prayer, God, answer hers.

God probably sees me like an impatient child, as when I told Jessica this morning that she had to wait an hour after taking her medicine before she could have breakfast. She wailed,

"I'll never eat again!"

I wipe my face and stare some more at the fire and think about something Jesus said in his Sermon on the Mount,

> "Ask, and it will be given to you;
> seek, and you will find;
> knock, and it will be opened to you.
> For everyone who asks receives,
> and he who seeks finds,
> and to him who knocks
> it will be opened.
>
> Or what man is there among you who,
> if his son asks for bread,

will give him a stone?
Or if he asks for a fish,
will he give him a serpent?

If you then, being evil,
know how to give good gifts
to your children,
how much more will your Father
who is in heaven
give good things to those who ask Him!" (Matthew 7:7-11)

I'm not sure I understand how tragedy can be a good gift. Strangely, Hollywood helps illumine me.

Bored of sitting by the fire, I put on a video—The Robe. Edd and Jessica, drawn by the story, join me. In one scene, Tribune Marcellus (Richard Burton), after going half crazy from crucifying Jesus and being touched by His blood and death robe, meets a singing paralyzed woman from the village Cana. She tries to convince him of Jesus' power to heal lives.

"Then why did He leave you as He found you?" Marcellus asks.

"I used to wonder about that myself," she replies. "He could have healed my body, but then it would seem natural for me to laugh and sing. He did something far better. He chose me for His service, so all like me may know that their misfortunes need not keep them from joy in His kingdom."

Marcellus, a Roman in a leather uniform, stares at her for awhile, shakes his head, and replies,

"What you believe is beyond all reason."

Yet, at the end of the movie, Marcellus walks joyfully to his death, sentenced by the Emperor for being a Christian. His bride walks next to him, holding Jesus' robe on her arm.

I also get inspiration from literature.
Mary Shelley was an amazing woman. The daughter of a

well-known feminist, she lived in England in the nineteenth century and married the poet Percy Byshe Shelley. Mary had several miscarriages and still-born children. None of her children who survived birth lived to adulthood.

She kept getting pregnant and giving birth—to deformity and death.

No wonder she wrote a gothic novel called <u>Frankenstein</u>.

A contemporary author named Marilyn Heavilin had three babies die—one of SIDS at a few weeks old, and a pair of twins shortly after birth. Then her teenage son was killed by a drunk driver. She wrote a helpful little book called <u>Roses in December</u> and worked with "The Compassionate Friends," a support group for bereaved parents. Marilyn's son is a friend of mine. I've met her and heard her speak.

Someone once came up to Marilyn and said,

"I am so glad to meet you—the one chosen by God to suffer so much."

Marilyn didn't feel special.

I've heard the sayings "No Pain Is Wasted" and "Don't Be Afraid of Tomorrow; God Is Already There."

But, come on, I'm really not all that much into pain. I'd rather learn about joy.

I have my own rose story:

"Rosebud in November"

Shortly after my last miscarriage, Edd, the kids, and I took a walk down by our beautiful mountain lake. Part of the lake, by "the village," is landscaped with lawns that reach to a wooden fence lined with rose bushes. On the other side of the fence is a sandy white beach, and the lake curves beyond that in little bays and open water.

I was amazed that the roses were still blooming in November, red against their overgrown green leaves and thorns. I stopped to examine one tiny, perfect bud. It was velvety to touch, perfectly formed, with dewdrops inside its symmetrical folds. I picked it and took it home, thinking,

That's what a miscarriage is like. The bud is picked before it can bloom...

At home, I put the rosebud into a small glass vase and set it on my bedroom dresser. Then I made a big mistake. I forgot to shut the door. When I went back into the bedroom that evening, I found the vase tipped over, water all over the dresser top, and the rosebud missing.

It didn't take me long to figure out that one of our [stupid] cats got to it. Sure enough, I found it in pieces under the barstools. "D. C." (Dumb Cat), our young black male, was pawing one petal. Another petal was hanging out of his mouth.

I almost laughed. My sentimental little rosebud, the symbol of my last miscarriage, was eaten by a cat!

I also get inspiration from music. It makes me cry. As you know, I hate crying. It always makes me feel miserable, messy, and upset.

The Psalms are songs—poetry set to music. King David of Israel is my favorite psalmist. The Psalms are a mix of suffering and joy—a call to God for help, and a hymn of thanks. David was not afraid to ask God questions or complain when things weren't going right. Yet David had faith that God would make everything right somehow. All you have to do is read Psalm 23.

My favorite contemporary musician is Steven Curtis Chapman. Steven is not just a good musician who plays the guitar, piano, and sings. He is not just a songwriter with a dozen CDs out over the last fifteen years. His songs are like poetry, written from his life experience, blended with scripture. They always speak to my heart:

> "The morning finds me here at heaven's door
> A place I've been so many times before
> Familiar thoughts and phrases start to flow
> And carry me to places that I know so well
> But dare I go where I don't understand
> And do I dare remember where I am

I stand before the great eternal throne
The one that God Himself is seated on
And I, I've been invited as a son
Oh I, I've been invited to come and...

Believe the unbelievable
Receive the Inconceivable
And see beyond my wildest imagination
Lord, I come with Great Expectations..."

I get inspiration from the Apostle Paul and the Apostle Peter's letters, too. Paul seems pretty much perfect to me, but Peter had his struggles. He was the one who denied Christ (three times!). He was the one who walked on the water to Jesus, then started sinking when he noticed the wind and the waves.

I found Peter in an art gallery. My friend Sarah has a lovely mountain art gallery. It's like a little bit of heaven, filled with soft music, peaceful landscapes, animal portraits, mothers with children, angels, and chocolate mints. It reflects Sarah's own gentle personality. We buy pictures from Sarah when we can. Sarah sells my books.

One picture we bought from Sarah is a tall painting of Peter sinking into the waves. Jesus stands on the water above him, reaching down with one arm to pull the terrified man up.

The caption reads:

"Why did you doubt,
Oh you of little faith?"

I feel so much like Peter. Surely I should see that Jesus loves me and will not let me drown.

Eleven

Making New Grooves

I used to ask my college English students "When did you first discover that life was out of your control?"

For me, that answer is "When was it ever in my control?"

If you read <u>Crossing the Chemo Room</u>, you know that my father shot himself in front of my mother and me on Christmas day before I turned five. My brother was just a baby. You also know that my mother became an alcoholic, dragged my brother and me across America in our old Dodge car, and then died when I was 24. My brother, who had been in jail and mental institutions, disappeared a few months later.

Christmas didn't start out well for me. It still brings an emptiness for family that is not there. Edd feels this way, too, since both his parents are gone (his mother Ruth died of lung cancer six weeks after I took her to the Emergency Room that night). Edd has siblings and cousins, but they are not involved in his life or are only there to cause problems.

Christmas can bring out the worst in families. I remember how my mother used to get melancholy and drink wine. This year, down in the valley, Edd's brother goes on another drinking binge, and neighbors call the police and Child Protective Services.

Linda, who is eleven now, doesn't want to live with her father anymore. She's sick of the mess the apartment is always in, the chaos of her life, and her father's drinking. Her brother

Chris (age nine) is terrified of losing his father. Neither child has lived with their mother for three years. She lives in another county and drinks even more than their father does. The Family Court ordered her to go into a thirty-day rehab before she could be alone with her children. She refused. The dad lets her take the kids anyway, just to have a break.

Why do some people even have children?

It's been nine months since we moved my in-laws out of our valley home and into an apartment that we found for them. They have been surviving mostly on welfare. I wrote this last spring when we moved them out and cleaned up after them:

"Sea of Clouds"

This morning we descend from our mountain to our old home in the valley. We gradually leave the trees and sunshine and dark blue sky, passing into the smog layer that presses down on the valley in shades of orange and brown. I clench my teeth as Edd drives on crowded freeways, too close to other cars.

We turn on our old dirt road and enter the open chainlink gate where I used to hang Christmas lights and a wreath. Edd's brother is still living here with his children. We're making them move out by the end of the month. They've trashed the place and can't pay us nearly enough to cover the mortgage.

We need to sell our former home.

Today the land is green after recent rains. The two and a half acres have a short covering like English turf. Wildflowers of small blue, yellow, and pink blossoms cluster among cast-away toys, plastic bottles, and stray pieces of firewood.

As soon as the car stops, Jonathan runs to hug Tina the dog (who will need a new owner soon). We rescued Tina, a black Boarder Collie, from the pound just before Jessica was born. She was supposed to be a gift for Grandma Ruth who didn't want her.

Jessica heads for the pine tree that has grown taller since we first moved here when she was a baby. When I had cancer,

Jessie would run out to the tree and try to reach its lower branches. Then she learned to pull herself up and sit on those lower branches. Now she climbs all the way to the top and perches in the crown. Behind her, between the branches, I can see sky, a few clouds, and the distant mountains.

I used to live here and look up at those mountains.

Edd goes to talk to his brother and start boxing up stuff to take to the dump.

I hesitate to get out of the car, knowing what kind of work awaits me. My in-laws have not cleaned the house in a year and a half. They just throw stuff on the floor. I'll be sorting through the giant pile in the kids' room and carting out a dozen large black trashbags full of junk. I'll be using whole bottles of industrial-strength cleaner, scrubbing filth off cabinets and toilets and tubs until my shoulders ache. I'll be climbing into dark recesses where rats have left droppings. I'll be scraping black spots off linoleum floors.

I drink some of my bottled ice tea and think about Chris and Linda who will be arriving home from school soon. Linda will scream when she sees our car from the bus stop. She'll run to her cousin Jessie who will give her the big silver box that holds her birthday present. Chris will show Jonathan his new Hot Wheels cars and ask to play Nintendo. I'll watch the children sing and play and chase each other across this land and think how they don't know what's coming—a small apartment in a local town, a new school, and life with their alcoholic father.

My brother-in-law goes to the local church sometimes, or he sends the kids (the church is just two fields away). Or well-meaning church members pick them up and take them. Sometimes my brother-in-law stays home alone while the kids are at church—and drinks. A dose of Nyquil can send him into a diabetic coma. When the kids come home and find him drunk, they call friends from church who rescue them temporarily.

My brother-in-law hasn't gone to AA meetings. He thinks they're a waste of time.

The children's mother doesn't visit much. When Linda calls her, she sounds drunk on the phone. The oldest brother,

P.C., is now seventeen. He has a part-time job after school and on Saturdays. He stays away as much as he can and won't be moving to a two-bedroom apartment.

Sick of these thoughts, I put on my facemask and gloves and begin emptying boxes on the patio. Not used to the heat, I take off my sweater and roll up my sleeves. I sort through the dusty collection of old tools and garden supplies and hardware which Edd collected and intended to use but which remained on the patio. The mess isn't entirely Edd's brother's fault.

But the yard could have been cleaned. I ask the kids to grab garbage bags and help me pick up the stray items that hide in the fields. I tell them I'll gather the many pieces of wood that have rusty nails sticking up from them. It's amazing that Chris or Linda haven't stepped on one and ended up in the Emergency Room.

As I toss board after board into a pile, I get angrier and angrier. Edd's brother and P.C. could have done this. I've accomplished more in an hour with four children helping than two men have done in the past year and a half.

It's the Vacuum Factor. If someone doesn't do his job, he creates an empty space that must be filled by someone else. Someone who has her own job to do ends up doing two.

I return to the patio to sort through a couple of book boxes that we didn't mean to leave there. The boxes have some rat droppings and a lot of dust on them, so I take each book out, one at a time, and wipe it off. When we get home, I'll put the books on the deck and spray them with Lysol before bringing them into the house.

I go into the house only to use the bathroom. I don't want to see the thick layer of grime on everything and the pile on the floor that hasn't been swept in months, next to the catbox that desperately needs changing. The smell makes me want to run back outside.

I used to live in this house and take care of it. I used to like this place.

Edd takes a load to the dump—the first of many. Our pickup truck is piled high with rusty chairs and an old sofa and rotted-out tables. I take a break to drink more tea. When Edd comes back, we wash ourselves as much as we can in the filthy bathroom, then go meet our friends Leslie and Dennis for dinner. We bring Linda and Chris along. Linda's eleven now and on the brink of puberty. Her long black hair curls down her back, and the crystal cross earrings and matching pendant I gave her shine against her bronze skin. I hope womanhood doesn't bring her too much pain. I hope she doesn't follow the path of her mother. Chris is almost nine and small for his age. I hope he doesn't follow the path of his father.

Why does family have to be a curse? I'm glad Edd and I escaped our families' curse.

I see four cousins before me. Two are from a world of drunken parents, filthy houses, hand-me-downs, and yelling through the night. Two are from a well-kept home among the mountain trees, from ice rinks—cold and quiet in the mornings—and classical music, and parents who kiss them into bed at night. They all four sit together at one end of the long table in a restaurant. They giggle and chat and squirm. Linda laughs loudly, and I wonder if she's afraid of the future. As the oldest child at home, she'll have to watch her little brother after school and deal with her dad's drunken spells when he passes out on the couch or doesn't know where he is because he's having a diabetic attack.

Wouldn't a foster home be better?

After dinner, we drop Chris and Linda at Marvin's house—a friend from church. As we pull into the suburban driveway, the four cousins finish singing a song they learned at church, their voices blending well.

"Take my life and use it, Lord," they sing. "Guide my feet into your steps."

Chris has second thoughts about the toy he gave Jonathan. Linda doesn't want to get out of the car. She hints at coming up the mountain to stay with us. We tell the children to follow us up the sidewalk. Marvin lets us into his cheery living room where the basketball game is playing. We sit down in his overstuffed easy chairs and talk for awhile, learning things Edd's brother doesn't tell us—like the time P.C. had to call 911 because he couldn't wake his father up one morning.

I decide to bring the cousins up for two weeks at Eastertime. I'll get used to having them sleep in the downstairs bedroom and telling them to pick up their clothes and put them in a drawer. I'll buy four new color-coordinated plastic cups, one for each cousin. I'll make them put the cups neatly on the clean countertop after a meal. I'll feel sad when the cousins leave and I have to wash the cups and put them away in the cupboard.

Edd and I thank Marvin for his hospitality and say goodbye. Exhausted, we drive back up the mountain by eleven. Our two children fall asleep in the back seat, lulled by our low voices, the long day of running across fields, and the car's motion. Edd drives; I look out my side window which faces the mountain slope. We've just broken above the cloud layer. It stretches out across the vast valley, a sea of clouds illumined from beneath by a faint yellow glow of city lights.

I feel like I'm in an airplane looking down. The stars shine above the cloud layer. I roll down the window. The air is different up here, cool and fresh and filled with evergreens. Even the gravity and air pressure are lighter.

I feel like I've left Hell for Heaven. For I was a child like Linda, trapped in a poor, single-parent, alcoholic, messy home. I was called White Trash. God called me out of there. He redeemed me to the mountains, brought my feet to the heights.

I could step out and walk across those starlit clouds.

In-laws aren't my only bad Christmas memory. Four years ago at Christmas, I had that miscarriage at four months—little baby Michael whom we buried in the yard. You can bet I was depressed. This Christmas, I have pretty much given up on the idea of having another baby, so I drink strong tea and eat chocolate. The chocolate helps me feel better, but after I eat it, I think about how I need to lose weight.

"You look sad," my friend Cherie tells me when I arrive at her house out of breath, my arms full of stuff, and my two kids trailing behind me.

"It's Christmas," I reply.

"You need new grooves in your brain," she advises cheerfully as she takes packages out of my weary arms. Despite four kids, Cherie has decorated her house with fresh pine branches and has spiced cider boiling in the kitchen. I stare around me, then back at Cherie. Her cheeks actually look rosy, and her blue eyes sparkle. I try not to envy her. She nods her head which makes her short brown hair bounce while she goes on to explain,

"You have these deep grooves carved in your brain by past experiences and emotion—your father's death, the miscarriage—all that makes you feel sad. You need to make new grooves—happy experiences, joy..."

I pause, considering her words.

"Yeah. You're right," I admit, wondering where these new grooves will come from. "I do want to know more about joy."

"Then go for it!"

After my visit with Cherie, I realize that I do love the Christmas season. In our new mountain home, late at night when everyone else is sleeping, I like to sneak upstairs and look at all the decorations. The tall glass doors, bordered by dark wood, are outlined in tiny white lights. The long metal railing by the stairs is entwined with a garland and more white lights. The fireplace mantel has red, pink, green, blue, yellow, and orange lights spiraled with red bows and greenery. Above it stands the nativity scene (we have only three wise men and 2 angels), the Menorah, and a painting of Mary kissing baby Jesus. The heavily adorned tree stands in the corner by a large window. I like to stand in the middle of the room, surrounded by all the lights like stars reflecting in the windows and glass doors. I look up through the corner window and see the moon, almost full...almost too beautiful to look at, like a living creature in the night sky, like an unborn child...

I pick up a strand of lights and hold it, thinking about my two young children sleeping downstairs, their faces angel-like in the hushed hues of their green nightlight. And Edd sleeps in our corner bedroom which overlooks the forest now covered with snow—and the stream that winds down over ice and rocks.

I have so much to be thankful for. Why do I feel depressed?

I wrap the strand of lights around me. They glow like something alive, like Christmas. I believe that anything can happen. I remember Christ's promise:

"I am the light of the world."

And I begin to make new grooves.

I bring flowers to my adopted Jewish mother, Gloria. She is tall and thin with red hair and glasses.

"Thank you so much for the flowers. They look so Christmasy!" she exclaims, hugging me tightly. She invites me in, and I notice her Avon boxes and catalogues spread about the living room (she sells me face lotion; I have no time for makeup).

"How are you doing?" she asks as she makes me tea with cookies. She admonishes me not to go out with wet hair (I never have time for blow-drying) and offers to bring me chicken soup because I have a cold. I notice her beautiful green glass Menorah on the fireplace mantel.

"Edd bought a silver one for our anniversary," I tell her as I stir my tea.

"I'm going to my daughter-in-law's for Christmas," she confides. "We celebrate Hanukkah and Christmas."

I look surprised, and she smiles.

"That's cool!" I reply. "We like to light the Hanukkah candles."

I keep the children busy. First, they march with the ice skating club in the annual mountain parade. Then, Jessica does her figure skating program to "The Blue Danube" music, in the Christmas on Ice show at the rink.

After that, we have a big party in our new house all decorated with lights. Thirty of our friends come, bringing their children. Cherie and her husband Bill are there, as well as Steve Smith and his wife Mary. Steve is a musician like Edd. He even looks like Edd—big, a little chubby, bearded, jolly, wearing a red plaid "logger" shirt. They can sing and play guitars together well past midnight if given a chance. Mary is like a sister to me, though we look nothing alike (she is short, with short dark hair, and I'm a tall blonde). Mary will listen to my problems and pray for me.

My best friend is Mary Pat. We are so alike (crazy writer types), and we can tell each other "like it is" and fight like sisters. Mary Pat has red hair and hazel eyes—very Irish-looking. She and her husband Randy stay late, sharing leftover Christmas cookies and hot spiced cider with us, their daughter Kaley happily playing with Jess and Jon downstairs as we four adults chat around our dining table.

Randy is a local science teacher, and five-year-old Kaley knows all the names of dinosaurs.

We are blessed with mountain friends.

Jessica and Jonathan sing in the choir for Christmas Eve service. Jessie has her first solo, the third verse of "O Come, O Come Emmanuel." She steps bravely up to the mic, her red and green dress blending into the background of the giant Christmas tree that fills our church's three-storey window.

Ask me to speak to any size crowd, and I will. But don't ask me to sing.

The most amazing event this season is Jonathan being baptized two days before Christmas. Big sister Kristen comes up to witness this event. She sits next to me in the long wooden pew while Edd goes up with Jonathan. He holds our little boy as they stand in the big baptistry, waist-high in water. Jonathan, only six and a half, looks so shy and small up there in front of our big mountain church. But he is able to recite his memory verse and tell how he "prayed with Mama" to ask Jesus into his heart. The pastor stands next to Edd as Edd bends down and dips Jonathan's little body under the water. Edd speaks the words,

"I baptize you in the name of the Father, the Son, and the Holy Spirit."

After the church service, Cherie comes over to me and says,

"See, you're making new grooves."

Twelve

Knocking on Doors

I've been writing a sequel to my new fantasy novel <u>Selah of the Summit</u>. I call it <u>Selah's Sword</u>. Ten years after the slavegirl Selah left the power of The Craft and the hot valley to journey toward freedom on the Summit, she is back in the valley. She has lost Micah to a strange disease which she herself survived. Even their daughter Evergreen was stricken, and Selah has left the sick child in the care of her friend Muriel while she searches for a cure. As she is in the valley searching, she rescues other slaves, constantly battling darkness and exploring deeper tunnels beneath the Keeps. Selah is swordsick. Her fellow soldiers tell her to return to the Summit for rest, but she is obsessed with freeing as many slaves as she can—as she explores a labyrinth of doors.

I feel like Selah. She is obsessed with opening doors wherever she goes. She keeps hoping that she will find that cure behind one of the hundreds of doors she has beat on with her fist or smashed down with her sword.

I've thought of a third Selah book (to make it a trilogy), <u>Selah and the Stars</u>. In this final adventure, Selah returns to the Summit and goes through The Portal, the doorway that leads to a new Zone above valley and mountains—the stars. She pursues Regan who is trying to spread The Craft to other worlds. Thus I turn fantasy into science fiction.

I sit in front of the computer and stare at some items on the screen. All my manuscripts are neatly labeled as word processing documents. Parts of all of them exist on my website. But only three of them are actually published in small, high-tech paperbacks with color photos on the cover.

I'd like to give them all a voice and a form—a solid, three-dimensional shape you can hold in your hand. They are my other children, unborn.

Maybe I am not meant to sell a lot of books and be in the public eye. Edd, the kids, and I are sheltered here on the mountain, in our house surrounded by trees. If my books became well known, that would change, wouldn't it? Do I really want to be part of the showmanship that goes along with promoting books and speaking to groups and the media? Do I want everyone to know the details of my life? Or was that the reason I wrote to begin with—so that people can read my story? Is there a safe place between fame and anonymity?

Maybe the timing isn't right yet. How much longer will it be? Some writers die before their work is widely known. Many writers never live to see their books loved by millions. Many writers have lived tragic lives, addicted to drugs, going insane, dying young, living in poverty.

I pause in typing on the keyboard and walk into the living room. There is a painting high on the living room wall. It is called "Iron Man," and it stares back at me: grim and silent, an old soldier, painted by Rembrandt in dark hues contrasting with gold from his helmet and armor. His face looks gold, too, creased by shadows, wrinkles, and frowns. His black, mysterious eyes seem to follow me.

He has seen his battles. Would he give up?

God can open any door He wants. He owns them all.

I wander back into the computer room, place my fingers back on the familiar black plastic keys, each marked with a white letter, and pray,

Lord, help me to write the story and make it beautiful.

The year after I went through chemotherapy, I attended my first writer's conference and wrote this:

"The Envelope in Liza's Hands"

I walk into the Case de Real convention room at San Diego State University and sit down on the floor. I'm late, as usual. I took my time walking across the campus where I got my B.A. and M.A. degrees in English, where I met Edd, and where we got engaged. I took my time in getting coffee and muffins at the complementary breakfast bar. Part of me must not want to attend the San Diego Writers' Conference.

There must be three hundred hopeful writers in this room, most at the tables. They look through their conference schedules and get out their pens, ready to take notes. I feel like a reporter come to write about the "behind-the-scenes" conference as I sit and watch one person and then another, wondering who I will meet and why.

The conference organizer introduces each speaker (editors, agents, successful writers) one at a time. I can't see the head table from my position on the floor, so I wander out to the lobby. I pour another cup of coffee from the dispenser, add creamer and sugar, and sit down on a couch. A man in a navy sports jacket writes something in his leather-bound notebook. Two middle-aged women in dresses sit near each other and chatter. I stir my coffee and wait for the first lecture, "How to Get an Editor's Attention."

After the lecture, which basically boiled down to "get an agent," I wait to confer personally with the speaker, Liza Dawson, Senior Editor of Putnam House, New York. She specializes in women's nonfiction. Several other women stand in front of me, so I turn to chat with a fellow conference attender, a pretty woman with curly brown hair and a business-like appearance.

"So, what do you write?" I ask.

"Actually, I'm just starting out as a literary agent. My name is Jeannette."

And thus I meet a possible ally. But I don't get to speak to Liza yet.

Later in the afternoon, after attending other lectures and a luncheon, I find myself sitting across from Liza. I just got myself some coffee, so I brought her a cup too. She is enduring another group of hopeful female writers who cornered her on the patio to share their ideas, projects, and lifelong dreams.

One woman, about fifty, with long, grayish-blonde hair, sits to Liza's right. She tells her about a nonfiction project that deals with the Baby Boomer Generation. Liza patiently listens as the woman outlines her thesis. The woman, dressed in a purple pantsuit, fidgets with her purple ink pen. I notice the crystal dangling on a purple string from the woman's neck. The Purple Lady. I wonder if her house is purple too.

"Well, I think your project might be hard to sell," Liza replies honestly.

The Purple Lady, undaunted, explains further why her project should be published. Liza repeats herself and suggests that the woman return to writing fantasy novels.

The Purple Lady writes down a few comments in her notebook. The summer sunlight slants through sycamore trees, across the tiled patio, through the wrought iron railing, and toward my eyes. I look up from my own manuscript that I've been holding with tense fingers. Liza and I are alone now, sitting opposite each other in lawn chairs.

"Here's my manuscript, <u>The Chemo Room</u>," I say, feeling like I'm imposing. She has accepted manuscripts from several of us already.

"Tell me about it," she suggests.

I speak, wondering if I am making sense. She listens, a tall woman in a loose black pantsuit over a white silk blouse. Her medium-length hair is dark brown, like her eyes. She's my age, with topaz glasses and a bracelet of translucent stones like hardened honey.

I listen to her words, good advice like "Know what other authors write about your topic. Who is your favorite non-fiction writer? To whom would you compare yourself?" and "Change your title. Don't go for just the cancer approach. Try for a broader base."

As she speaks, I think how ordinary and astounding she is, with her black leather sandals over knee-high stockings and her brown-leathered watchband holding time to her wrist.

She doesn't once look at her watchface.

My writing life has led to this point, across from Liza Dawson in the afternoon sunlight at San Diego State University. And suddenly I feel like bursting into tears as she speaks to me. All those years of writing, the college degrees, the months of chemotherapy, each word spelled one letter at a time—and the exhaustion and the rejection letters and the computer keys tap, tapped into midnights—condensed to these few minutes between us as I endeavor for something clever to say.

Maybe Edd is right about the vanity of self-promotion. Maybe all this effort just isn't worth it.

Liza and I pause as sunlight illumines the air between us, sparkling on a bit of dust, a fallen leaf, an insect's transparent wing. I wonder if she hears the sobs in my mind, unvoiced. Why do I want to cry? For myself? For the Purple Lady? For all the hopeful writers who will never get a book published by Putnam House? For cancer patients whose story was never written?

Words seem fragile, now, as I pass my manuscript to Liza and say, "Thank you."

She reads so many pages. Will she throw my papers into the hotel trash bin? I wouldn't blame her. She's got luggage to carry back to New York.

Will she remember me, that I brought her coffee and spoke of cancer and Christ?

Jeannette, my possible new literary agent, breezes toward us.

"If you don't hear from me, send me your manuscript again," Liza leans toward me and says.

I remember her advice about sending manuscripts through an agent. Jeannette pulls up a chair beside me.

"So, if I give my manuscript to Jeannette, and she mails it to you, you'll read it, right?"

We all laugh a moment, and I stare again at my manuscript wrapped in a tan-colored envelope that Liza holds fast in her hands.

Thirteen

Island of Healing

Linda and Chris, the cousins from the valley, came up for a visit last weekend. We contacted Child Protective Services, but they're not doing anything. Too often, children who really need to get out of a bad situation stay in it, and families who homeschool their children are harassed.

I broke my ankle while Chris and Linda were visiting. At two in the morning, a family of raccoons playing outside our bedroom window woke Edd and me up. Edd went back to sleep, but I couldn't. So I went upstairs for a snack and some late-night T.V. When I was done, I carried my empty box of Fig Newtons down the dark stairs and missed the last step that leads to the den where Linda and Jessie were sleeping on the couch.

That will teach me to hold onto the rail.

I broke my left ankle badly (I don't do things halfway). I even started shaking, going into shock. But, since it was two in the morning, I just hobbled into bed, huddled under the blankets, and somehow slept until morning.

Maybe it's just sprained, I hoped unrealistically.

I was able to hobble around on it Sunday morning (Edd left early to lead the church music), getting beds made, kids ready, and breakfast served. But it had swelled pretty badly, was starting to turn purple, and hurt a lot, so I drove the kids to church and got the pastor's wife to drop me off at the E.R. just down the street.

Not long after the x-ray results, I discovered that my bone had actually separated about an inch, and I would need surgery, a metal plate, six screws, and thirteen staples to put me back together. I would stay overnight at the hospital because they wanted to monitor my pain. After seeing the physical therapist and learning how to use crutches without putting any weight on my left foot, I would be released Monday afternoon.

It was kind of fun being in the hospital. Edd brought all four kids to visit me, then drove Chris and Linda back to the valley. I got to sleep as much as I wanted. When I was awake, the nurses took good care of me, bringing me all the juice I could drink and giving me Demerol shots (hey, I'll take pain killers anytime).

Not until I got home and found myself stuck in a stair-filled house with crutches did I start to feel sorry for myself.

Then Nina came to visit. She brought my late Christmas present: green embroidered towels for my upstairs bathroom and a gold-toned angel frame that I was going to use for the picture of our new baby that we lost. She hardly looked like she was five months pregnant with twins, in her trim snowflake sweater and jeans. She told me she was going to have a girl and a boy and hugged me, saying in her Russian accent,

"I pray for you, Lonna."

I didn't cry then—not until after she left. While Edd took the kids to the rink, I was left alone in the house with the headset phone, my pain medicine, a glass of water, and the T.V. remote in close reach on the table beside the sofa where I lay with my leg iced and propped up on pillows.

God, I cried, why does Nina get twins, and I get a broken ankle?

My cast is fiberglass and light, but I'm tired of hobbling around with it covering my left foot as I bear all my weight on my right foot or the crutches. Muscles ache that I didn't realize I had, especially in my arms and chest.

From the sofa, I stare out through the wood-trimmed glass doors of my mountain home.

The afternoon sunlight slants down onto clusters of pine

needles, cedar boughs draped like lace, and silver fir branches spread wide like a canopy. A gray squirrel jumps from branch to branch, and a funny little bird walks straight down a treetrunk. A red-tailed hawk glides on air currents above the treetops. The wind blows everything, making a symphony of light and color in the three-dimensional zones of the forest.

The American Indians were right about modern man being separated from nature. Vast cities swarm below this mountain, reaching in a maze of freeways and houses to the sea. How much could it help some of those people to come to the mountains and stand in the silence and sunlight, with time enough to think about their lives and where they are going?

My next door neighbor Kathy moved up to this mountain recently, leaving behind a gang-infested neighborhood. Her daughter had a baby at sixteen and was shot dead in a drive-by shooting when she was seventeen, leaving the little girl for Kathy to raise. Then, trying to cope with his sister's death, Kathy's son got in trouble with drugs and the law.

"I wish I had moved up here sooner," Kathy tells me.

Yesterday she brought her son up here to live. I see him out the window. He's a tall, slightly chubby twenty-four-year-old with a shaved head and baggy clothes.

"He's a lost soul," Kathy says.

I pray for him, that he will find peace and a purpose in these mountains.

I read Psalm 72, a psalm of Solomon the Wise, son of David. I knew Solomon wrote Proverbs, but I didn't realize he also wrote a psalm.

> "Give the king Your judgments, O God,
> And Your righteousness to the king's Son.
> He will judge Your people with righteousness.
> And Your poor with justice.
>
> The mountains will bring peace to the people,
> And the little hills, by righteousness.
> He will bring justice to the poor of the people;

He will save the children of the needy,
And will break in pieces the oppressor."

At first glance, this is a psalm about the mountains and the peace found here. But the trees themselves cannot solve all life's problems. If you look closely at this psalm, you can see that it speaks about the Messiah—and the peace and justice He will bring.

It's not enough to be among nature. You need to know the Maker.

I'm not the only one who has suffered physically. I have had friends who live in wheelchairs. One was a wild truck driver named David, who, after a bad accident in his rig, found himself a quadriplegic with limited use of his arms and hands. He had to depend on his wife for many of his daily activities.

Then I met someone even more physically challenged:

"Ron's Chin"

Recently I met a man named Ron Heagy. He is a more severe quadriplegic than David was. He speaks to groups, especially high school students, and tries to encourage them to face life's problems and overcome.

"Are you happy?" he asked my church group. He paused while we thought about that, then continued, "You know, your attitude is everything. Let's face it: life is a problem. You've either just gotten out of a problem, are in one, or are going into one. It's how you <u>face</u> the problem that matters. Your attitude. Look at me. I could hide in my room and feel sorry for myself. I'm paralyzed from the neck down. What's your excuse? Are you paralyzed from the neck up?"

The audience laughed. I thought, as I sat there thinking about my fifth miscarriage, *I am paralyzed in my heart.*

Ron spoke about people getting out of their comfort zone

and doing something wonderful with their lives. He told the well-known story of Jesus and the storm, how He walked over the water toward the wave-tossed boat full of His disciples, how Peter left the relative safety of the boat and started walking on the water toward Jesus.

Ron has accomplished amazing things. He started an outdoor camp where physically challenged people can go. He writes and even paints with his mouth. Just before he came up the mountain to speak to us, he had an accident in his wheelchair. Helpless, he fell to the side and cut open his head. Now that's a problem.

I had to admit that night, as I sat there still brooding over my miscarriage, that I can learn something about joy from a man in a motorized wheelchair—that he moves by a control stick he operates with his chin.

When we lived in the valley, I knew a woman in a wheelchair. She was a paraplegic, so she had strong upper body strength and could get around well in her sporty wheelchair. I wrote a story about her:

"Kara's Chair"

At our last "park day" for my homeschool association, I talk to Kara as we sit at a picnic table. I met her earlier this year and chatted lightly with her, but today we really talk.

She is a beautiful woman with long blonde hair, a symmetrical, clear-complexioned face, blue eyes, and a trim figure. Her white shorts contrast against her tanned legs.

She is also in a wheelchair.

After a few introductory remarks, I look at her and ask, "Were you in a car accident?"

"Yes," she replies immediately, uninhibited about discussing her story (she's been asked before). "It was right after my honeymoon nine years ago. I was driving my husband's truck, alone. I lost control, and the truck jumped over the curb and went down a hillside. It flipped several times. I wasn't wearing my seatbelt, so I was thrown out onto the ground."

"Nobody saw me go over the edge. An off-duty paramedic noticed the tire tracks soon after it happened. He used his radio to call for help. A helicopter took me to the hospital. I was bleeding internally. I almost died. Later the doctors told me that they had to do open heart surgery. They didn't tell me about my spine until I recovered from the surgery. I wouldn't believe them until I saw the x-rays.

"The break was bad. I realized that the doctors were right—I wouldn't walk again."

"Were you a Christian then?" I wonder.

Kara grins. "Yes. So was my husband."

Kara's daughter runs up to us. She looks like her mother—tall, with graceful arms and legs and long, blonde hair. She's eight years old.

"Mom, may I have a drink?" she asks.

Kara reaches to the table and hands Phylicia a bottle of water.

"So you had your two children <u>after</u> the accident," I observe.

Kara laughs. "Yes. I had just gotten out of the hospital—after five months. I was still getting used to the wheelchair when I found out I was pregnant with Phylicia. I had Shane three years later. During the pregnancies, things were a little awkward but not that bad. I have good upper body strength. The wheelchair always seemed perfectly natural to my children. They never knew me another way. I still like giving them rides."

Shane comes to visit us and report that he has to go to the bathroom. Phylicia takes him to a porta-potty at the park's edge.

"I like the church I go to now," Kara tells me as she watches her children in the distance. "It's the first church I've gone to where people don't come up to me and ask why I don't have faith that God will heal me."

"I've heard that line before," I admit.

"I know God can do anything. I believe it's His will for me to have gone through what I did and to be like this. I've grown in so many ways because of this wheelchair. I wouldn't change things."

"Wow!" I exclaim, wishing I could say the same about my cancer and the miscarriages.

"Don't get me wrong," she continues, leaning toward me. "It hasn't been easy. I didn't always feel this way. After the kids were born, for months I was terribly depressed. My husband finally told me that he could take all of what went with the wheelchair—but not the depression. I decided that I wanted my marriage to work, so I snapped out of the depression."

I stare at Kara for a moment.

After awhile her children return from the potty.

"Mom, can I have a ride?" Shane asks, eyeing the sloping sidewalk at the park's edge.

"Sure," Kara replies. Shane climbs on her lap, and Kara wheels past the picnic table quickly. Kara and her son zip past people and trees, big smiles on both their faces. Their laughter echoes across the manicured lawn.

"Noni"

I have always gotten plenty of exercise, eaten a diet high in fresh vegetables, breathed deeply, and taken my vitamins. Still I got cancer. While going through cancer, I discovered the world of herbs and other nutritional supplements. I take several herbs daily, and am especially fond of chlorophyll geltabs, green tea extract, grape seed extract, ginkgo biloba, spirulina (freshwater blue-green algae), echinacea, aloe vera juice, and flax seed oil. Herbs really can help boost your immune system, clear your brain, and keep your digestive and cardiovascular systems healthy. I got my cholesterol checked recently, and my doctor said I had one of the best levels he had ever seen.

Everyone wants to feel better, in one way or another. When I was in Kauai last summer, I was amazed at the emphasis people put on health and exercise. Kauai is called the "Island of Healing." If you've been there, you can understand why. Kauai is surrounded by ocean and island outdoor adventures, bright-colored flowers that bloom year-round, and a tropical environment of sea breezes, sunshine, rain, and 70-degree temperatures. They're also 2900 miles from any polluting continents.

At one resort, Jessica and I got up early to take a "Tropical Stretch and Energizing Class." It was a combination of a nature walk, exercising, and yoga. I felt chubby and out of shape next to the petite instructor whose boyfriend was in sports medicine. She rambled on about the importance of diet and deep breathing.

"This is the Noni tree," she pointed out on our walk. I stared at the medium-sized, bushy tree with broad leaves and green fruit that looked like small unripened pineapples.

"Its juice can cure anything from depression to cancer."

So that's what I'm missing, I thought, Noni.

But life is more than exercise, meditation, diet, herbs, and miracle fruits. One can even get into other things like magnetic fields, infrared light, lasers, and homeopathy. But no matter how much we take care of ourselves, accidents happen. We will die eventually. The fittest people on earth have perished in a car crash or dropped dead from a heart attack. And when we're so focused on our own health, don't we become self-centered? Shouldn't we risk a little contagious disease by reaching out to the sick?

Only Jesus can heal eternally. As the prophet Isaiah says:

"Surely He has borne our griefs
and carried our sorrows;
yet we esteemed Him stricken,
Smitten by God, and afflicted.

But He was wounded for our transgressions,
He was bruised for our iniquities;
the chastisement for our peace
was upon Him,
and by His stripes we are healed." (Isaiah 53:4-5)

᪥

When I returned to my mountain after staying in Kauai, I realized that I live on an "Island of Healing" also. This island is not surrounded by water, but by millions of people in their cities, thousands of feet of rock, a vast canopy of sky, and a sea of clouds that roll in white waves beneath the mountaintops.

But, like Selah, I can't stay here on my Summit. I've got to go down to the valleys, touch the people living there among gangs and drugs and depression. Right now I'll be doing that only with my words as I lie on the sofa, my casted foot propped up on pillows while I type on my laptop and pause once in a while to look through glass doors to the forest. The sunlight is getting higher in the treetops as evening approaches. The wind swirls around leaves and branches, bringing a message. It's the same wind that blows over cities and continents, oceans and islands. Maybe it blew all the way from Kauai.

I finished <u>Selah of the Summit</u> in Kauai, sitting at a table by a window that overlooked Hanalei Bay. Behind the bay rose the mountains, covered by rain clouds and waterfalls.

Fourteen

Lord of the Rings

Since I broke my ankle and have to wear a cast and hobble around on crutches, I've been housebound a lot—especially when it snows. Crutches don't work well in the snow.

I've been feeling sorry for myself and asking God questions like "Why have you brought so much trauma to my life? Don't you love me? Am I one of Your lesser children?"

I've got a new perspective on things. When I sit at the bottom of my red-carpeted stairs and look up, the slope seems so much higher and more intimidating than when I was able to stand and climb them. Life is a Quest, even if the journey is inside my house.

When I go to my mountain church and sit in the front, I stare at the red carpet below the altar. Sunlight shines down on it, through the tall stained glass window, making rectangle shapes of yellow, green, and blue. I'd like to lay face down on that pattern and ask God,

"Why did I have five miscarriages?"

By the time I stand before God in person and ask that question, the answer won't matter.

I stare down at my crutches under the pew and see them lit up with a bluish silver light. It looks beautiful, like the glow around Frodo's sword in <u>The Lord of the Rings</u>. God healed me of cancer, and these crutches are only temporary. I can still fight.

"Lord of the Rings and Harry Potter"

When I was teaching college English, one of my students once said, "It must be terribly boring to teach literature." Obviously that student had not explored the power of words, the adventures of the imagination. Every English teacher I have known has lived life rich in adventure—even a man named J.R.R. Tolkien, who was Professor of Medieval Studies at Oxford University in England. He used to go out into the woods near his home and dance with his wife under the moonlight. And he wrote some books about hobbits who live in a place called Middle-earth.

I love <u>The Lord of the Rings</u>. I was a teenager when I first read <u>The Hobbit</u> and the ring trilogy (<u>Fellowship of the Ring</u>, <u>The Two Towers</u>, and <u>The Return of the King</u>). The only thing I was sorry about after I finished those books was that I could not read them again for the first time.

I remember thinking how long Frodo's journey lasted. I felt tired just reading about it. Tolkien's words put me in the wasteland of Mordor, thirsty and hungry and lame, my eyes steadily fixed on Sauron's burning tower. I was impressed by Sam's loyalty as he supported the heavy-hearted Frodo. I admired Gandalf who used his wisdom to fight evil. I wanted to meet the elves—tall and graceful and wise—guardians of forest and rivers, healers, oldest of all the races.

I wanted to date someone like Aragorn, heir of the king who cut The Ring from Sauron's hand. Aragorn, strong and trustworthy, was the best of the young race of Man—the Chosen One who would bring peace to Middle-earth.

Most of all, I liked Frodo, simple and brave. He was a hobbit from the peaceful Shire, a farming country filled with parties and food. Frodo never studied witchcraft or asked to go on a quest. He didn't want the task given to him: carry the evil Ring to Mount Doom and throw it into the fire where it was made.

The <u>tone</u> of Tolkien's writing lured me into his world, his vision of the heroic tale, his own creative soul. The descriptions, the settings, the character development all complemented the graceful sound of Tolkien's poetic sentences and Elvish language.

I read almost everything of Tolkien's, including the history of Middle-earth, <u>The Silmarillion</u>. I read Tolkien's authorized biography. I read about how Tolkien was friends with C.S. Lewis, another of my favorite writers. I read just about everything C.S. Lewis wrote. I got a Master's degree in English and taught college for awhile. I thought I had a handle on the idea of heroic literature. But there is more to <u>The Lord of the Rings</u> than can be learned in a college class.

Tolkien never considered <u>The Lord of the Rings</u> as children's books. All of the characters are adults. Tolkien was a Christian and considered his books to be religious and Christian in nature, though he did not make them allegories (as C.S. Lewis did in his fiction). Tolkien saw the Gospel of Christ as the Real Story, the true heroic tale of God's sacrificial, redemptive love for us. Tolkien believed that all of our invented stories are mirrors of the Real, coming from the part of us that longs for our lives to mean something, that longs for a relationship with God and God's people. Tolkien shared this idea with Lewis, who was an atheist at that time. Lewis thought about the possibility that in The Gospel all our heroic tales somehow come true. A few days later, C.S. Lewis became a Christian.

The idea of God is woven subtly into Tolkien's books. In <u>The Silmarillion</u>, Tolkien writes about The One who made the universe and everything in it, who guides and protects the events and people of Middle-earth.

But instead of drawing long quotes from the books, let's look at the first movie which captures Tolkien's vision.

I am a fan of Peter Jackson's films. I've seen <u>Lord of the Rings: Fellowship of the Ring</u> several times. Before it came out on DVD, I went with Andrea Smith, a seventeen-year-old high school student, babysitter of my kids, and editor for my books. We sat together, commenting on crucial scenes and memorizing lines. She thought Frodo was cute. I thought

Legolas, the elf archer, was also cute. We debated on whether or not Gandalf the Wizard is a sorcerer or a wise man (the word "wizard" can mean either).

I admit that the film isn't perfect. Peter Jackson changed a lot of things from the book. Some of the changes were good, such as the fast pace of the film (the book is very long). Some changes are not good. The wizard battle scene was overdone (it wasn't even described in the book). Jackson could have spent less time showing orcs' heads getting lopped off and more time developing characters. Tolkien wrote very little about orcs and battle scenes. He spent far more time describing the natural settings of Middle-earth. I guess Jackson used violence because some people say "cool" when the bad guy gets stuck with an arrow between the eyes. But violence should not be so much a focus. Jackson could have shown it less directly (a bloody sword instead of a stab in the face, for example). A lot of people would rather look at Frodo or an elf, or the beautiful scenery of New Zealand with mountains stretching to the sea.

But let me state the reasons I love the film—and why I think it presents a Christian rather than a non-Christian world view.

I do have some problems with the fact that Gandalf is a wizard. This could lead someone toward witchcraft. Even though Tolkien did not use "wizard" in the witchcraft sense, it could still be a problem if a person obsesses over <u>The Lord of the Rings</u>. We must remember that the story is, after all, not absolute truth—but one man's vision. At least Gandalf is a humble wizard. He does not know everything. He treats Bilbo and Frodo with kindness and respect, encouraging them to do the right thing with The Ring but not forcing them. When Bilbo refuses at first, Gandalf shows his well-controlled power, saying:

"Do not take me for some conjurer of cheap tricks."

We never see Gandalf mixing herbs into a cauldron or reading from a witchcraft book. When he does speak in a special language, it is Elvish.

After Bilbo finally abandons The Ring to his unsuspecting

nephew Frodo, Gandalf doesn't even dare to pick it up. He lets Frodo do that—then hide it safely away. Gandalf leaves to research the historical records because he doesn't know enough about The Ring. When he returns to The Shire, he sadly explains The Ring to Frodo, after Frodo takes it from the fireplace and sees the fiery letters on it:

> Three Rings for the Elven-kings under the sky,
> Seven for the Dwarf-lords in their halls of stone,
> Nine for Mortal Men doomed to die,
> One for the Dark Lord on his dark throne
> In the Land of Mordor where the Shadows lie.
> One Ring to rule them all,
> One Ring to find them,
> One Ring to bring them all
> and in the darkness bind them
> In the Land of Mordor where the Shadows lie.

Gandalf knows how much trouble Frodo will face if he carries The Ring to its doom. His wrinkled eyes express his sorrow, but he knows that only hobbits can perform the task. Gandalf gives Frodo a companion—his nosy gardener Sam—and the two begin their journey. Gandalf leaves in another direction, to consult with the wizard Saruman, who has become an ally of the evil Ring-maker, Sauron.

Gandalf begins to suspect this when he enters Saruman's tower of Isengard and warns him not to look into a Seeing Stone, for "you cannot be sure who is watching on the other side." Saruman does not listen to Gandalf. The two wizards do battle with their staffs, and it is obvious that Saruman's power comes from the evil Sauron while Gandalf's comes from a totally different source.

The book shows this better than the film. In "The Council of Elrond" chapter, Elrond and Gandalf condemn "sorcery." Gandalf explains that Saruman has become evil because of his pride and lust for power and that "It is perilous to study too deeply the arts of the Enemy, for good or for ill" (page 345, Ballantine Edition).

Before he escapes from Saruman's tower, Gandalf explains that The Ring was made by the evil Sauron who is like a lidless eye wreathed in fire, always watching. The Ring will corrupt anyone who wears it. It must be destroyed. One cannot compromise with evil.

"There is one Lord of the Ring," he warns Saruman, "and he does not share power."

Gandalf is rescued by the King of the Eagles and rejoins the two hobbits at Rivendell. Others join the quest to destroy the ring: Aragorn, the human heir of Gondor, the elf Legolas, the dwarf Gimli, Frodo's hobbit friends Pippin and Merry, and Boromir, another human.

Gandalf leads The Fellowship of the Ring over the snowy mountains. Gandalf doesn't want to go through the dark Mines of Moria, but the blizzard forces him. Once inside the mines, he has a talk with Frodo who misses the sunny Shire.

"I wish the ring had never come to me," the hobbit says. "I wish none of this had happened."

"So do all who face such times," Gandalf replies. "But that is not for them to decide. All we have to decide is what to do with the time that is given to us...There are other forces at work in this world, Frodo, besides that of evil. Bilbo was meant to find the ring, in which case you also were meant to have it."

Gandalf has a sense of God's protection and sacrificial love. He shows this best when he faces the demon at the bridge of Khaza-dum.

"I am a servant of the Secret Fire," he says as he stands on the bridge and blocks the path. "You cannot pass." The light from his staff crystal glows like a halo around him, and the demon falls into the pit, dragging Gandalf in after him.

Other characters in the film show compassion, wisdom, and courage.

Arwen, the elf princess, is a good addition to the film. In the book she is barely mentioned. In the film Arwen is sent to rescue Frodo. She shows an awareness of God as she carries the wounded hobbit across the river toward Rivendell. After the Black Riders have been swept away by a flood, she stares at Frodo who is gasping for breath.

Tears come to her eyes as she prays:

"Whatever grace is given me, may it pass to him. Let him be spared. Save him."

One of my favorite characters is the beautiful blonde Galadriel, Queen of the forest Elves at Lorian. She is wise and can read people's minds. Though Gimli the Dwarf calls her a sorceress, she is not one. She does not follow witchcraft books, mix spells, ride a broomstick, or wave a magic wand. Instead, she asks Frodo to look into a water mirror.

"What will I see?" he asks, afraid.

"Things that were, things that are—and some things that have not yet come to pass," she replies mysteriously.

Frodo looks into the silver bowl. He sees the ruin of The Shire, the trees uprooted and turned to black wasteland, and Sam being led away in chains.

"This is what will happen if you fail," she tells him.

In the book, Galadriel discusses the mirror.

"This is what your folk would call magic, I believe; though I do not understand clearly what they mean; and they seem also to use the same word for the deceits of the Enemy," she says (page 468).

Even Galadriel doesn't want to use the word magic.

Frodo offers her The Ring, and for a moment she considers it, turning into a terrible warrior queen. But then she becomes herself again and joyfully says,

"I have passed the test! I will diminish and go the west and remain Galadriel." She turns and kisses Frodo on the forehead, telling him, "Remember that even the smallest person can change the course of the future."

When she sends the rested Frodo and his company up the river in Elvish boats, they are wearing forest pins on green elvish cloaks. Before they leave, Galadriel gives Frodo a glowing crystal vial.

"May it bring you light in the darkest places, when all other lights go out," she promises.

And so the little hobbit travels on with eight companions. One will die, and the others will be scattered while he and faithful Sam continue toward Mordor. Frodo will remember what Gandalf told him: "All we have to decide is what to do with the time that is given to us."

Tolkien believed that God gives us our time. Near the end of his life, he told a little girl that a person's highest purpose is to learn about God, serve Him, and be thankful.

Now let's contrast <u>Lord of the Rings</u> with the Harry Potter world by J.K. Rowling. I admit I am biased here (aren't all humans biased?). I don't like the books—or the films, which follow the books pretty well. From the first chapter of the first book, <u>Harry Potter and the Sorcerer's Stone</u>, I was turned off by the <u>tone</u>. The book, set in modern England about a witchcraft school for children, puts down those who don't practice witchcraft. They are called unimaginative, boring, cruel "Muggles."

Rowling claims she did not originally mean for the Harry Potter books to be for children. If this is so, why are the main characters children?

One reason I don't like Harry Potter is he isn't as kind or honest as Frodo is. Harry Potter and his friends hate Muggles or anyone else they consider their enemies. They are out for revenge.

"'I'll get him,' said Ron, grinding his teeth at Malfoy's back, 'One of these days, I'll get him—"

'I hate them both,' said Harry, 'Malfoy and Snape.'" (page 196)

The very non-magical Frodo is not looking for revenge. He just wants to do his job and go home, staying out of Sauron's way as much as possible.

In <u>Harry Potter and the Sorcerer's Stone</u>, Professor Snape turns out to have protected Harry from evil instead of cursed him. Still, Harry makes no apologies for the way he felt about his teacher.

At the end of the book, Harry has revengeful plans for his Muggle family. "<u>They</u> don't know we're not allowed to use magic at home. I'm going to have a lot of fun with Dudley this summer," he says (page 309).

Rule-breaking is rewarded in the book. Harry and his friends constantly break school rules and get away with it. Rule-breaking even brings adventure. When he flies on his broom against the rules, Harry is rewarded by being put on the Quidditch (flying soccer) team, something that rarely happens to a "first year" student.

Harry and Ron lure their friends into their rebellion, especially Hermione, a star student. "Hermione had become a bit more relaxed about breaking rules..." (page 181).

Stealing is also encouraged. When Harry's Quidditch team wins, "Fred and George stole some cakes and stuff from the kitchens." (page 227). Harry constantly lies to cover up his rule-breaking. Even Professor Dumbledore, the Headmaster at the school, says "The truth. It is a beautiful and terrible thing, and should therefore be treated with great caution" (page 298). Dumbledore also says (concerning Harry's parents' death) "After all, to the well-organized mind, death is but the next great adventure" (page 297).

Harry Potter is more of an anti-hero than an epic hero.

Violence is clearly described in the Harry Potter books. In the first book, an evil wizard kills a unicorn and drinks its blood in a moonlit forest. The wizard also possesses another man's body and then kills him. The sequels (<u>Harry Potter and the Chamber of Secrets, Harry Potter and the Prisoner of Azkaban,</u> and <u>Harry Potter and the Goblet of Fire</u>) get darker than the first book. Violent deaths and scary battle scenes appear more often. Ghosts and goblins populate Harry Potter's world, and humans are possessed by spirits.

Correct me if I'm wrong, but in all the Potter books, I see no concept of God. Society is purely secular. The characters solve their own problems. There is no Higher Force guiding or protecting them. True, Harry Potter's world is full of adventures, interesting characters, humor, imagination, and surprises. One reviewer said that the only people who don't love Harry Potter books are boring Christians.

What is witchcraft? Webster defines it as "the use of sorcery or magic." Though Harry Potter shows witches and wizards as "good" or "bad," is witchcraft ever good? What is the purpose of studying witchcraft? To battle bad witches and wizards? Doesn't the power from witchcraft come from one source?

Professor Snape tells the students in his potion-making class:

"I don't expect you will really understand the beauty of the softly simmering cauldron with its shimmering fumes, the delicate power of liquids that creep through human veins, bewitching the mind, ensnaring the senses...I can teach you how to bottle fame, brew glory, even stopper death" (page 137).

J.K. Rowling is no Christian. She studied witchcraft to make the books more believable. Exactly what she believes has never, to my knowledge, been pinned down. I saw her interviewed for A & E Network's <u>Biography</u> series. She claimed that her books don't lead children into witchcraft.

"Children understand that they're just fiction," she stated.

If that's true, why do so many children send Rowling letters asking if they can go to Hogwort's School of Witchcraft and Wizardry? Why have kids been known to look for Platform 9 3/4 at train stations? And why have brooms, potions, capes, wands, and crystal balls become popular items for sale at such places as Renaissance Faires? Witches use such things in their rituals. Visit any witchcraft store or website and see for yourself.

The fifth book, <u>Harry Potter and the Order of the Phoenix</u>, has just come out after three years in the writing. It is nearly 900 pages long and darker than the other books. One of the major characters dies. When Rowling was interviewed by Katie Couric on <u>Dateline NBC</u>, she said that she was very annoyed by people who accuse her of leading children into witchcraft.

"It's utter garbage," she stated. "Not one child comes up to me and says 'you turned me onto the occult. Let's go sacrifice a goat together.' I believe in God. I'm on their side."

If I were Katie, I would have asked her which God she

believes in. I've known children who have been turned toward the occult in part, at least, because of the Harry Potter books and the sense of power they bestow. Such a child might not go up to Rowling and admit this. Sacrificing a goat is an extreme part of witchcraft, not the subtle first steps.

"You believe that there is one God. You do well. Even the demons believe—and tremble!" (James 2:19).

If one believes in God, one does not necessarily serve Him.

Fiction is based, at least to some extent, on nonfiction. And children don't have the logical reasoning abilities or experience of adults. Children may see only make-believe fun in the books, but that does not mean there is nothing more there.

And what does the Bible say about witchcraft? Is it harmless? Or is it part of the dark force of Satan himself?

The Old Testament clearly states that one must avoid witchcraft, divination, and sorcery (see Exodus 22:18, Leviticus 19:26, Deuteronomy 13:1-11).

The prophet Samuel told disobedient King Saul that "rebellion is as the sin of witchcraft." (1 Samuel 15:23).

In the New Testament, sorcery is listed as one of the "works of the flesh." Those who practice it "will not inherit the kingdom of God." (Galatians 5:19-21)

I ought to know about witchcraft. I used to study it. I gave it up when I became a Christian. Christ's love, His death for me, and His resurrection power shine like a light into the darkness of witchcraft.

What a witch believes and what a Christian believes are opposites. Ouija boards, Tarot cards, and seances may seem like fun, but they are connected to a darker force. I can walk into a witchcraft shop and feel the dark power reaching out like an unseen hand. Witchcraft may seem like it gives power to its users, but it actually enslaves them. Like The One Ring, it corrupts all it touches, turning even good intentions to evil. If you do not realize this, you have never really dealt with witchcraft. Or you have been deceived.

"Satan can appear like an angel of light," The Apostle Paul

warns us (2 Corinthians 11:14). In Ephesians, Paul tells us that we have an enemy. He says that we must always be watchful and "put on the whole armor of God, that you may be able to stand against the wiles of the devil." He goes on to add:

> "For we do not wrestle against flesh and blood,
> but against principalities, against powers,
> against the rulers of the darkness of this age,
> against spiritual hosts of wickedness
> in the heavenly places." (Ephesians 6:12)

There is more to Harry Potter than harmless fun and children's literature. Go into any bookstore and see what is displayed with the Harry Potter books. You will find books on witchcraft and casting spells. On the Halloween when the first <u>Harry Potter</u> movie came out, my local mountain library offered a children's Harry Potter night, complete with witchcraft and wizardry lessons.

The Apostle John, in his first letter to the churches, warned of the spirit of antichrist that is in the world. The world eagerly listens to that popular voice because the world "lies under the sway of the evil one." John also said that Christians are not part of that world system. We are separate from the world, so the world won't listen to us. The line between Harry Potter and Christians is well drawn. Where do you stand?

I'm sure my objections are like a pebble tossed into the ocean next to a hurricane. J.K. Rowling's books, traditionally released at midnight to hordes of excited children wearing starry wizard hats and black-rimmed glasses, packed into bookstores to wait in long lines, have sold 200 million copies in 200 countries in 55 languages. The two films have made 1.8 billion dollars. Her books have made Rowling richer than the Queen of England.

If I met Jo Rowling, I would probably like her. As a mother of young children, I used to write parts of my books on scraps of paper at coffee houses. Jo and I even have daughters the same age, both named Jessica. Perhaps Rowling doesn't fully realize the power of witchcraft. And I do need to thank her for helping to inspire me to write my own Selah fantasy trilogy, my alternative to Harry Potter, a Christian view in which I show The Craft as an evil thing that enslaves people. Selah the slave escapes the hot valleys and journeys to freedom in the mountains. Along the way, she discovers romance, the beauty of God's creation, and the joy of bringing light back down to the darkness.

As a cancer survivor, I felt sad when I read the story in Time magazine about the little girl named Catie Hoch who died of a brain tumor shortly after her ninth birthday. I commend Rowling for emailing, calling the girl on the phone to discuss Harry Potter, and sending presents in the mail. But I wonder if Catie was given any real hope of eternal life.

As Jesus said when he raised his friend Lazarus from the dead,

"I am the resurrection and the life. He who believes in Me, though he may die, he shall live." (John 11:25).

Surely Christ's Good News of eternal life holds more power than Harry Potter ever found.

There really are monsters in this world. Harry Potter lures us toward them. Lord of the Rings shows us what they really are.

But don't take my word for all of this. Study the Bible. Put it to the test. See if the Gospel really is the Greatest Adventure. Maybe you'll find yourself on a Quest, clothed in armor, sword in hand, fighting the enemy.

But don't lose focus. Don't stay in the battle scenes. Keep your eyes on Christ. He has the final battle plans. He has already won. He, like the Returning King, will bring peace to Middle-earth.

For Further Reading

The Silmarillion and The Letters of J.R.R. Tolkien by J.R.R. Tolkien.

J.R.R. Tolkien: A Biography by Humphrey Carpenter.

Finding God in The Lord of the Rings by Kurt Bruner and Jim Ware.

The Lord of the Rings Official Movie Guide by Brian Sibley.

Tolkien's Ordinary Virtues by Mark Eddy Smith.

Harry Potter and the Bible by Richard Abanes.

Mere Christianity and Surprised by Joy by C. S. Lewis.

J.K. Rowling: The Wizard Behind Harry Potter by Marc Shapiro.

J.K. Rowling: A Biography by Sean Smith.

Conversations With J.K. Rowling by Lindsey Fraser & J.K. Rowling.

Harry Potter: Witchcraft Repackaged video by Loyal Publishing, 2001.

Internet Sources

http://www.family.org
http://www.thelordoftherings.com
http://www.thetolkienforum.com
http://www.tolkientrail.com
http://www.theonering.net
http://www.tolkienonline.com
http://www.tolkiensociety.org
http://www.jrrtolkien.org.uk

༄

I think about all this while I'm climbing my stairs, teaching the children, and leaning on my crutches at our big upper-storey window. The sky, even at night, is white with clouds, the full moon behind them, and new snow which covers the tall cedar trees. The trees surround our house like sentinels. They seem glad under their weight of snow which makes different patterns on different trees. The pines have clumps, the cedars broad fronds, and the fur trees boughs droop down like lace-covered arms. From the snowbank below, our house stands like a tower of wood and glass in the mountain forest. At midnight, when the clouds clear, the full moon shines directly down, shadowless, lighting up the white slopes like a fairyland.

And somewhere far away, Frodo and The Fellowship of the Ring trudge through a blizzard in a mountain pass.

Fifteen

Michelle and Me

I love ice skating—the silence of early morning when mist rises over the ice, the sound of blades cutting into the surface, and the wind in my hair. When I hold my arms up at my sides, palms down, I feel like I'm flying.

Before I broke my ankle, the kids and I practically lived at the rink. At first, we went just for fun and exercise. We would lace up our rented skates and wobble around on the ice, grabbing for the nearest sideboard. It didn't take me long to get my ice legs back, since I had learned to skate as a child. I began skating backwards, trying my crossovers, and doing a spin or two. My children, being closer to the ice than I was and less afraid of falling, soon learned to zoom around the rink like hockey stars.

Then they discovered figure skating lessons.

Now, four years and thousands of dollars later, the kids are aspiring future Olympians. I hobble on my walking cast and bring them to the rink. No longer do they use rental skates or the public rink (it didn't help that its roof collapsed). Now they train at the same rink as Michelle Kwan. Now we order $500 custom boots separate from $400 blades—unless I'm lucky enough to find good used skates. Jessica is getting taller, and her feet have hit an—ugh—growth spurt. Jonathan has little chubby feet, and it's hard to find small black figure skates (we tried hockey skates on him once, but he screamed for us to take them off because they had no toe pick).

Now the kids skate several times a week, have their own private coach, and take ballet, powerskating, and jump classes. We see Michelle Kwan three times a week when she's getting ready for a big competition. I gave her a signed copy of <u>Crossing the Chemo Room</u>, and she politely accepted it. I wonder if she'll ever read it...

We also see some of the other top world figure skaters like Sasha Cohen (U.S. Silver Medalist), Alexander Abt (Russian Silver Medalist), and Anthony Liu (Australian National Champion).

Before I broke my ankle, I learned my inside and outside edges, how to do a spiral, skate faster backward, and complete a better spin. But I wasn't about to throw myself up in the air and turn around a few times before landing back on the ice.

Then I broke my ankle and had to wear a cast for two months. That first month, in January, I hobbled around on crutches. One Monday afternoon, I somehow made it to the rink despite the recent snowstorm. I maneuvered my way from the car door, across the parking lot, and up the sidewalk that was covered with ice. When I got inside, Michelle Kwan looked at me and said, "Be careful."

She either thought I was crazy or a very dedicated skating mom.

"I didn't do this on the ice," I felt compelled to tell her. "I did it on my own stairs, at home. I hope this doesn't happen to you."

She smiled and turned to do her usual warm-up routine. I felt really dumb because the Olympics were coming up in a couple of weeks, and I had just mentioned the possibility of breaking a bone to our top American figure skater.

When the Olympics finally came, Edd (who makes the money to fund our figure skating madness) sat with me and the kids in our cozy mountain living room. The fireplace was blazing while snow fell lightly outside our big picture windows and landed on the evergreen trees. I propped my cast up on a pillow, hogging most of the sofa while we, like millions of other people, were glued to our T.V. set for way too long while NBC brought us too many commercials between their scattered coverage of The Games.

During the Opening Ceremonies, we cheered for the skaters from our rink—the ones we had seen week after week, practice after practice—who gave candy to our kids, sat with them for photos, and signed their skating boots. We watched as Sasha Cohen stood next to President Bush and handed him her cell phone. We watched Michelle wave and smile.

"I know how she feels," Jessica announced. "She's really wants to be treated like an ordinary person who just loves to skate."

We watched all the figure skating events, which NBC didn't usually start covering until 9:00 p.m. We endured all the switching back and forth between bobsledding, skiing, speed skating, and figure skating. We stayed up until midnight most nights and swore, when the Olympics were over, that we wouldn't watch T.V. for a month.

We cheered as Todd Eldredge (six-time National and World Champion) did his last Olympic long program—to <u>Lord of the Rings</u> music. I interviewed Todd once for <u>Blades on Ice</u> magazine. He seemed like a really nice guy who likes to golf in his spare time and support his local community by building a sports park.

We followed the Pairs Skating controversy, taped all the long and short programs, and finally discovered the surprising outcomes when the champions stood on their podiums to receive their medals.

We felt really disappointed for Michelle because she got a bronze medal and not a gold one. We could tell that she was disappointed, too, as she held back tears and stood there, poised, with a brave stare in the face of what she considered defeat.

When we saw her at the rink about a week later, she came in silently with her mom and dad. Estelle sat down in the chair behind me, and Danny went to get his customary cup of coffee while Michelle avoided the eager little skaters with pens in their hands.

I know that being third in the world isn't bad. I would love to be third in the world of writing. I started writing when I was four, probably about the age Michelle was when she laced up her first pair of skates. I would follow my grandmother around her big house and ask her what letters objects began with.

"What says 'toothpaste'?" I would enquire.

"'T,'" my grandmother would patiently reply.

"What says 'paste'?" I would quickly respond. And so the lessons began...

As you know, I wrote through my childhood—about my father's death, my mother's alcoholism, and my brother's disappearance. I wrote about the time my mother shut herself in her bedroom, refused to eat, and drank only rubbing alcohol. If I hadn't called 911, she would have died by morning. I wrote about finding the wine bottles hidden in her bedroom closet. I wrote about the times my mother drove a race car, galloped on a runaway horse, scuba dove in a lake, flew in a biplane—how she taught me to be daring and different and a little rebellious.

I had the perfect childhood for a writer.

Then I got my Master's degree, married, and had kids. I wrote through my cancer, keeping up my journal through surgery, chemotherapy, and nausea. I described how I lost the last strands of my hair and what funny things you can do with a wig. I shared how God, my husband, doctor, nurses, and friends helped me through the whole cancer experience.

I wrote with all my heart, as Michelle skates with all of hers.

I haven't made money like Michelle has. I haven't been offered a $50,000 advance or won the Pulitzer Prize. Like Michelle, I've set a goal for myself but have not reached it.

So I continue to write when I can find a free hour. I often bring my laptop to the rink, but it's hard to type when my fingers are cold. I sit with the other rink moms and dads and half watch my kids skate. I'm usually running late, so I get a seat a little further away from the heater. I bring my long "polar bear" coat with a scarf, gloves, one Ugg boot, and a thick blanket to cover my legs. It can get boring to sit and watch my daughter see how low she can go on her sit spin. Her long braid flies out behind her, woven with yellow and green ribbons that match her velvet skating dress. She goes so low that she collapses on the ice. My son wants me to watch everytime he does his toe-loop, and if he catches me chatting with another mom, he'll spray ice chips on me with his "hockey stop." Then he grins, showing his big dimple and his blue eyes and his wild, curly Irish hair.

The day at the rink drags on. I can't wait to start skating again (my doctor tells me I've got a few more weeks). I think it's more boring and exhausting to sit and watch than to get out there and skate. So I buy strong coffee. I ask the box office attendant for a new ice time schedule. I rummage through the lost and found bin to see if my kids left their blade guards or gloves. I sit back down, watch Jessie's coach strap her into the "fish hook" harness so that she can work on her axel, check out Jonathan flirting with a pretty blonde teenager in a skimpy black skating dress, and then start chatting again with the mom next to me. We talk about the edgy coaches, the bossy skating moms, how temperamental our children are, and the high cost of figure skating.

"No, I don't want to do that hard jump," Jessie will tell her coach. Then she complains that he's not pushing her enough when he says, "O.K., let's work on something easier."

Sometimes I'm too tired to chat with the moms. I just want to haunch over my steaming coffee and observe life at the rink. We are a kind of family. We see each other regularly and watch each other's kids for a session when we have to run to the post office. We comfort a fallen child who has just split her chin open on the ice, offer to fetch a bag of ice or a bandaid, and yell at each other when we're stressed. We discuss the weather, what's happening on our mountain, and — of course — the recent news in figure skating competitions.

Lately, Michelle has been in a better mood. She smiles when she walks into the rink, does her warm-ups at the near end of the ice, and chats with us locals. She signs figure skates.

She's got a new goal. She's training for the World Championships.

So what do a cancer survivor and a world-class athlete have in common? We don't give up. And we both love to skate.

Sixteen

Lord of the Dance

I finally got the cast off my ankle and am walking around. The metal plate and screws are still in the bone, and it aches at night, but I can start skating again.

I wake up at 6:30 on a Saturday morning. While Edd makes my tea, I sneak into the kids' room and open the window blinds. Both kids are cuddled up in a fetal position, under their rainbow blankets. Jessie opens her eyes first, usually a morning person. Jonathan keeps sleeping, his little mouth open, drool on his cheek. I go over and cuddle with him, kissing his cheek, feeling his curls against my face, annoying the heck out of him. He groans and turns toward the wall. I don't go away. I tickle the back of his neck. He tries to shrug me away and opens one eye.

"I don't want to go Power Skating," he moans, trying to pull his covers over his head. Jess is already pulling on her midnight blue velvet skating dress and shiny tan tights.

I love waking Jonathan up. It's a type of revenge for all those times he exhausts me.

We have cereal bars for breakfast and then pile in the car. Hopefully, it's not icy on the mountain—but it's always cold this early. We arrive at the rink which is nestled among pine trees. The sun is just beginning to shine on the tops of them, above the cold, deep shade in the forest. There aren't many cars in the parking lot, so Edd pulls up close to the door.

Jonathan, unusually silent, drags his skate bag to the bench while Jessica, who has put her skates on in the car, starts her warming up exercises. Edd sits down close to the heater, pulls a blanket over his legs, and grades papers for his college English class. I stuff Jonathan's chubby little feet into new leather skating boots which are cold and very stiff. It takes several tries, each time loosening the black laces more.

"I can walk on water," Jonathan announces, unblinking. "It's called <u>ice</u>."

I laugh and think, this is what makes a figure skater. I finally lace the boots up, put on Jonathan's red cap and matching vest, and make sure he's got his gloves. Without thanking me, he takes to the ice, stroking fast for someone so small.

I sit down next to Edd, placing my huge stack of bills, checkbook, sewing kit, the cow doll, and her severed arm that needs sewing back on, into a pile at my feet.

I look around at the other skating moms and dads. Some have brought stuff to do, like me, and some just sit there and watch their little skaters the entire time. One mom looks fresh and awake, her makeup done, her hair perfectly styled, and her clothes looking like she just got back from the city.

I think about my own appearance: no makeup, hair barely brushed, a faded green sweatshirt over black velvet stretch pants, and well-used Ugg boots to keep my feet warm. How does this mother have time to put on makeup? Well, she has only one little skater, I think.

My distracted thoughts quiet as I watch other skaters step onto the freshly smoothed surface which is covered with a thin layer of water. They advance in a ring from all directions, as if beginning a dance. They stroke in long, graceful arcs across the ice, their blades flashing silver as they cut trails of circles and curves, thin lines intersecting and separating—where before there were no marks.

The ice is like my life, I think. What was clean and new is marked upon, like penmarks on a clean white piece of paper or letters typed upon a blank computer screen.

These skaters are confident, used to the disciplined freedom of their sport. Their legs stroke faster as they lean against the curves. They balance out their arms like wings about to take flight...

The ice is like the life we each are given. What will we write across the surface?

"Would you like some coffee?" Edd asks me. I nod, my thoughts turning to practical matters. He brings me a steaming cup, and we watch the skaters and write or grade papers.

When the morning session is over, Edd and I wait for the kids to dry off their blades and pack up their skate bags. I think about the rest of the week: later this afternoon we'll come back for the Rec Session. Then, after homeschool, on Monday afternoon the kids do two skating sessions (one with their coach and one without), followed by Ballet Class at the rink dance studio. Then the same two skating sessions on Wednesday afternoon, followed by Jump Class at the same studio. Then more skating sessions on Thursday and maybe Friday. I may take a walk through the forest during some of those sessions—no point in just sitting and watching others exercise. Or maybe I'll skate myself.

This is what makes a figure skater, I think again. The kids finally have their skate bags packed, and we walk out to the parking lot together. We have parked next to the well-polished mom with the one little skater. Her vehicle is a brand new silver BMW SUV with a personalized license plate. Our vehicle is a ten-year-old, beat-up Subaru station wagon of uncertain color, covered with mountain dust and loose twigs. It even has a bunch of recylables in the back.

Edd gets into the driver's seat and turns on the heater. I open the back hatch, and aluminum cans start pouring out onto the parking lot.

My life is a comedy, I realize. I could do stand-up.

I'd talk about when I wrapped a red silk flower around the rearview mirror and suggested we call the car "Rose." The kids both immediately informed me that the car was a boy, and his name was "Hunter." Considering how I drive on mountain roads, I understood why.

Sorry, Rita, about the time I nearly ran you over when I

came around a corner and you were standing in the road and watering your bushes. You had to leap into them to get out of the way...

The kids and I try to pick up the cans as they fall, then shove in the skate bags on top of them (why don't those cheap white plastic bags stay <u>shut</u>?). We pile in the car, which is full of all types of junk, such as soggy breakfast bars, dirty napkins, and broken toys. We watch the skating mom and her well-groomed little girl climb quietly into their shiny BMW.

Well, we could outdrive you on these mountain curves, especially in the snow, I think as Edd pulls away first.

This afternoon Edd builds a rock wall in the yard while the kids and I return for another session. The polished mom and her daughter are not there.

This is a special afternoon—my first back on the ice. The winter snow falls in big puffs outside the rink windows. I stand and watch from the inside. We're early for a change, and the rink is almost deserted. While Jessica goes to a bench and laces up her skates, Jonathan stays outside and spins around as thousands of flakes fall on him. The sky is gray, the glass between me and the snow cold as I press my fingers upon it. I stare up at the source of the snow and see the patterns it makes as it falls downward: on the fir tree limbs, on the cars, on the picnic table, on the sidewalk. Jonathan, in the midst of the flurry, dances with the joy of a child. His red hood is soon speckled white.

I watch for a while longer then call him inside before he gets completely soaked. I plop down on the bench next to him and pull my white Jackson heat moldable Freestyle figure skating boots out of their black bag, where they have for too long been neglected. I love the look of a figure skate. I pick it up and admire the shiny white leather, the curves, the inside padding, the bronze eyelets that hold laces. And the blade—aerodynamic, symmetrical—glints in the light, making its stainless steel glimmer like silver. I tentatively pull the left boot over my left ankle, feeling the metal plate and screws, wincing against the pain...

But the pain doesn't last long—or maybe I don't notice it

anymore once I finish lacing up both boots and step toward the ice. Our rink, with no sides, is like a smooth frozen pond that you just step out onto. I stand at the edge of the recently smoothed ice, and hesitate. I always step out with my left foot first, and somehow it does not want to leave the solid ground.

I wish Edd were here and that he could skate with me. But he's got a bad knee and can't afford a skating accident (he's much more sensible than I). I imagine him lifting a large white rock, putting his sturdy back into it, and setting it in a neat straight row on our side yard by the dry stream before the snow gets too deep...

Anthony Liu, Jessica's coach (Australian National Champion, former Chinese National Champion) is the only one on the ice. He notices me standing there and offers me his hand. I accept, glad to grab onto something for that first step. I take the step, amazed that my feet do not fly out from under me.

Anthony remarks "this is Williams family private ice," and laughs, skating away to give Jessica a lesson. I take my first strokes. I feel like a newborn calf, then slowly build up my balance and speed. Cool air sweeps across the ice, and I smell the frost in it.

I will never forget how to skate. It feels wonderful, and I know that, as long as I can skate, my health must be pretty good.

I swing my inside and outside edges wide as I stroke in curves and then skate backwards and do a spin. I catch my reflection in the mirrors at the rink's far end. Wearing my new bright yellow Polartec jacket and black pants, I look like a giant bumble bee. For a moment I feel awkward, wondering how a chubby, round, fuzzy bee with small translucent wings could possibly fly. But that thought doesn't stay long as I glide past the mirrors and catch up to Jessica and Jonathan. They smile, glad to see Mom on the ice again. They stay with me for awhile, and then Jessie starts her lesson with Anthony. We are the only four people on the ice this snowy December afternoon.

I think Heaven must have an ice rink and fresh-fallen snow.

Jonathan holds my hand for awhile and then easily skates past. For awhile I skate alone, losing myself in the strokes, thinking with my feet. Soon I'm dancing to the music from the rink CD player—a fast song with a good beat.

I feel like Selah of the Summit as I lean my head and arms back, look up, and say,

Thank you, thank you!
to the Maker of the Mountains,
Lord of the Dance.

Seventeen

I Could Have Done More

I've done a few book signings. But I'm not a good salesperson. Here is an example that happened three years ago:

"How Many Names?"

Today I return to The Little Professor Book Company in the valley for a book signing of <u>Crossing the Chemo Room</u>.

I leave the mountain early, taking Jessica and Jonathan with me—along with my new friend Mary Hughes and her five-year-old daughter Dolly. We drive down from snow and cold to a wide, green valley. We drive past the road where we used to live on two-and-a-half acres. We drive to the bookstore where I had a booksigning for <u>Our Mothers, Ourselves</u> on Mothers' Day, 1996, when I was going through chemo.

I step back into another life.

I'm fifteen minutes late, as usual (I hate wearing watches; they're like a band of slavery). Mary leaves me to browse through books, get a cup of coffee, and sit down in a stuffed leather chair by the fireplace (she doesn't get much of a break from kids either). Jessica takes the younger two to the train in the children's section. A good reader now, she will gather an armful of books to read to Jonathan and Dolly.

I set down the extra books I brought, on the table prepared for me. The manager put out some nice fliers, a potted plant, and a bottle of water. I sit down and wait to see who'll come.

A grandmother, who drove a long way to buy my book for her grandson who has lymphoma, walks over. She asks me to sign her grandson's name on the first page.

Denise Hilts arrives. She hands me an envelope with "Lonna Williams" scrolled across the top. It holds the article she wrote in <u>The Press-Enterprise</u> two days ago—about me and <u>Crossing the Chemo Room</u>.

She gives me a hug.

"Next time you're in town, call me, and we'll have lunch," she says.

"Thanks for coming by," I reply, signing her name in a copy of my book. "And you really should come up the mountain to visit us."

"I'm pretty busy at the paper these days, but maybe, when I get the time," she states, looking a little stressed. As I watch her open the glass door of the bookstore to leave, I remember that her mother died of breast cancer two years ago.

Other people, having read the article, arrive. Many are buying books for family members or friends who have cancer. One is a cancer survivor of several years who doesn't buy a book but leans over the table and congratulates me on my survival. I smile back at him. A college student in her twenties tells me she just found out she has breast cancer. She's going to the same support group I used to attend.

"Say 'hi' to Lori," I tell her. "Dr. Schinke told me she's still leading the group. It must be as wild and crazy as ever!"

The college student nods her head and buys a book. She mentions she's keeping her own breast cancer survival journal.

She leaves, and I get up and walk around for awhile, flipping through the bestsellers and magazines. Jonathan comes up every once in a while, waves a book in front of my face, and asks me to buy it. He's just learning how to read...

Mary shows me a book about menopause. Jessica and Dolly decide to change into each other's clothes in the ladies' bathroom. Mary and I make them change back.

Then a woman arrives, wearing a thick blue jacket. Her dark hair is short, and she has round glasses and a round face with a nice smile.

"Hi, Lonna," she says. She asks me questions, and I get a blank look on my face as I desperately try to remember who she is.

"See, my youngest is seven now," she says, pointing to the dark-haired child beside her.

"Oh," I reply. I still can't remember her. Is she from our old church? College? Where?

"What name should I write in the book?" I lamely ask as I hold my green pen above it.

"Becky," she replies.

I still don't remember who she is, probably because I'm not seeing her in her usual setting. Then she mentions that "the office has been busy lately with flu season." A glimmer of memory returns.

"My sister died last year of breast cancer," she finally says, tears starting to fill her eyes.

I realize I'm talking to Becky Ing, wife of Dr. Ing, my children's first pediatrician.

"Oh! I'm so sorry!" I say, standing up. I walk around the table and hug her. She starts sobbing in my arms, clinging to me like I'm a life saver.

I remember the day, three years ago, when I took Jessie to the doctor's office. I found Becky, the doctor's young wife who always seemed so strong, sensible, and "together." She was sitting at the computer in the front office, tears streaming down her face as she read an email.

She just found out that her younger sister, who had been battling cancer for years, had taken a turn for the worse.

I hugged Becky then, too.

"I remember that your sister and her husband adopted a child before she died. I'm glad she was able to do that," I say, coming back to the present and still holding on to Becky.

"The little boy is three now. His father brought him out to California to visit us this Christmas," Becky explains, dabbing at her tears with the tissue Mary brought her.

"That's nice that your sister left a child as a heritage," I ramble on, reaching for words. "It doesn't matter that the child is not her own flesh and blood."

Becky starts to cry again.

"Your sister is in a better place," I comfort, patting her shoulder. "No more suffering. No more cancer."

Becky looks at me, trying to gather her sensible doctor's wife and office manager self around her again.

"Thanks for reading my manuscript three years ago," I tell her. "The book is a lot better now after you marked it for corrections."

We chat for awhile about me selling our valley home and having a garage sale. Becky suggests I send fliers to the office. I invite her to come up and visit us in the mountains.

"Yes, that sounds nice," she says, her eyes looking away from me for a moment. I give her one last hug, and she picks up her book, holds her daughter's hand, and leaves. Mary sits down at the table next to me, and we consider Becky and her loss in silence.

The afternoon continues. A few more people come and buy my book. As I near the end of my book-singing appearance, another mother hands me a book and asks me to write her son's name in it. My eyes blur with tears as I write the name, wondering

how many names could be written?

"Why I Give Away My Books"

Though I have bills to pay, I'd rather give my books away. Why do I do that? I know it's not good business sense, but I hate to ask people for money. It's more fun to give a present, free and unexpected, than to figure out sales tax. I'd rather just hand over my small, shiny blue book with its high-tech cover and the photo of me and the kids, a year after chemo, hiking in the Canadian forest. Or my <u>Like a Tree Planted</u> novel, my first published book, with a photo of my teenage daughter Kristen posing in a futuristic silver vest under a eucalyptus trees. Or my newest, <u>Selah of the Summit</u>, the fantasy adventure story with a Canadian waterfall on its cover. I like to give the fiction books to children and teenagers.

I give <u>Crossing the Chemo Room</u> to cancer patients, mostly adults. There are so many of us. Everywhere I go, I meet those who have been touched by cancer.

In Canada, in December, we escaped California to rent a cabin by a frozen lake. Most of the resort was vacant, but three cabins down from us were John and Yvonne from Calgary. They brought their big orange cat with them on a month's vacation. The day after New Year, Yvonne was scheduled for surgery to remove a little liver cancer.

She was terrified, but when she met me in the resort's lobby, she seemed inspired that I was a survivor.

"You look too good to have been through cancer, "she said.

I tried to give her my book, but she paid for it with Canadian money.

Yvonne and John didn't want to leave their cabin by the frozen lake. On New Year's Day, they wandered through the resort grounds, past snowbanks, on walkways quickly covering up with new snow. The puffy flakes fell all around them, blending in with Yvonne's white fur coat and hat. John, tall and thin in his brown jacket, carried the orange cat in a blue pet transporter.

They looked like lost souls trying to find a path.

That's why I give my books away.

Even if I could afford to give all my books away, I would probably still feel like I haven't done enough:

"I Could Have Done More!"

"For to this you were called,
because Christ also suffered for us,
leaving us an example,
that you should follow His steps." (1 Peter 2:21)

The Apostle Peter knew about suffering. When he was an old man, Roman soldiers bound his hands and led him toward a cross to die. Peter, feeling unworthy to die as Jesus did, asked the soldiers to turn the cross upside down, and they did.

It's easy to feel joy when you are healthy and your life makes sense—when you have a loving family, comfortable home, meaningful job, faithful friends, lots of cool techno-stuff, and trees surrounding you. But real joy goes deeper than feeling, remains with us through pain, loneliness, and poverty.

Mother Teresa understood suffering as she worked among the poor people of Calcutta. She preferred their company to wealthy dignitaries who asked her to come and speak. Once a rich man sent a limousine to fetch her to a meeting. She refused to ride in the long white car, seeing, perhaps, the homeless children she could have sheltered briefly upon the plush red seats.

Stephen Spielberg understands suffering. He shows this in his film <u>Schindler's List</u>—a painful movie to watch because it is so true.

The film's ending is especially powerful. The Jews Schindler rescued from Hitler during World War Two gather together to present Schindler a gift—a gold ring made from the fillings in their own teeth and engraved with Hebrew. Schindler—well dressed, reserved, and tall—stands beside his expensive automobile. He picks up the ring and stares at it, speechless. Then he drops the ring, bends to retrieve it, and awkwardly places it on his ring finger. Tears come to his eyes as he weeps,

"I could have got more—I didn't do enough!"

He points toward his car and laments, "This car—why did I keep it? Ten people by that."

"You saved eleven hundred Jews," his trusted accountant reminds him.

"You have no idea how much money I wasted," Schindler replies, shaking his head.

He takes off his lapel pin and grieves,

"This pin—two people—at least one, one more person..."

Schindler collapses to the ground, sobbing,

"I could have got one more person, and I didn't, I didn't..."

The Jews, men and women, try to console him with their embraces as he continues weeping.

Billy Graham agrees with Schindler. I saw a T.V. interview Larry King did with the famous preacher. King seemed impressed and perplexed by Graham, leaning toward him, listening intently to Graham's answers.

"Do you think you've done as much as you could do in God's service?" King asked.

Billy looked at him for a moment before replying.

"No. I always think I could have done more."

Eighteen

Growing into their Feet

When I was going through cancer, my daughter Kristen was a teenager. She moved to Washington state with her father, and I missed her terribly. I was also angry at her. She had a choice where to live, and she abandoned me when I needed her...

I wrote about that in <u>Crossing the Chemo Room</u> (never cross a writer). After she read the book, Kristen complained,

"Mom, you made me sound like The Evil Daughter."

I realized she had a point. I also realized that I had gotten over my anger, and that I needed to write a more balanced story about her. She has grown up a lot—like a puppy grows into its feet. She's twenty-four now and very clear about what she wants to do. After getting married to Jeremy, the Christian carpenter, she hopes to be a missionary to Mexico with him. They're planning on staying in San Diego for awhile first and will probably have a few children.

"We'll still do things with you, like go to the Renaissance Faire," she assures me when I sound depressed about her upcoming wedding. I imagine we will still share experiences together.

Kristen and I have always shared lake experiences. This is for you, Kristen, my Lady of the Lake:

"Canim Lake"

A year after I had chemo, we took a vacation to British Columbia with Kristen, to celebrate her graduation from high school. My hair was growing back all curly and short like Jonathan's. We hiked in the great Pacific Northwest rainforest, and Kristen took that famous photo of me, holding onto a small evergreen tree, that became the cover of <u>Crossing the Chemo Room</u>. (Edd had decided to stay at the lodge and fish that day, or he would have been in it.) I wore Edd's white coat and stood with one hand on a fir tree, the sunlit forest around me like a picture frame. Jonathan (almost two) sat in his blue backpack and picked a leaf off my shoulder while Jessica (almost five) stood in front of me as I dangled my sunglasses beside her.

One afternoon while Edd fished on the pier with the lodge owner and the little kids played on the swings nearby, Kristen and I canoed up Eagle Creek, a river that flowed into Canim Lake. We passed a fallen aspen tree that a beaver was gnawing before it slapped its tail on the water and swam away. A little further down, we passed the beaver's house of sticks. We paddled against the current, getting caught in dead pine trees by the banks, discovering it's easier to go <u>with</u> the water's flow.

We turned around and found calmer water at Eagles' Cove. For awhile we drifted and watched a pair of loons. Then we saw an eagle swoop down from a tall spruce on the far side of the cove, its six-foot wing span skimming across the water as it headed for the pier where Edd has just released a fish. It's head glowed pure white in the sunlight, and it uttered a high-pitched cry as it grasped the fish in its huge yellow talons and flew back to its waiting nest.

"Well, this is real mother-daughter time," I said as we set the paddles across our laps, facing each other.

"Yes," Kristen replied. "We have to do this again."

Then we prayed together as water lapped against the canoe hull and the wind moved locks of hair near our faces. Kristen's face, delicate and thin and not yet blown completely into womanhood, still bore some freckles around her nose. Curly tendrils touched her shell-shaped ears.

I'll miss you, I thought, holding back tears.

ॐ

"Hendrix Lake"

As our Canadian vacation neared its end, Kristen and I explored another lake together one overcast afternoon. The lodge owner's wife told us about it.

"Hendrix Lake lies at the gateway to the real wilderness," she said from her post behind the lodgedesk. Her shoulder-length auburn hair bobbed as she spoke in a kind of hushed tone. "It used to be a mining town, abandoned twenty years ago. A developer tried to revive it, but only a handful of families live there now, since it's so far from everything. It's grizzly bear country. A local guide takes rich hunters out after the bears—in groups of six men. They camp on the land; the guide provides all the equipment except guns. Ten thousand dollars for a week. Once the guide shot a grizzly out of a tree. When he went to check it, it attacked him. His gun jammed, so the guide used it as a club. The bear lost, but the guide has scars all along one side."

"Wow," I said as I ran my finger along the map she had given me. The lake itself was not even on the map, but I saw Mount Hendrix clearly marked. Beyond it, the dotted (unpaved) road curved farther north and then west, past places with no towns next to them and which had names like Horsefly Lake.

Kristen and I packed the little ones in the car, glad the drive would be only about half an hour over a rutted dirt logging road. I took pictures of trees along the way: dead trees at the base of a clear-cut hill, old growth lined tall on both sides of the road, a valley of newly planted saplings sloping toward Hendrix Mountain.

Gee, these photos will be great for my website and a new edition of <u>Like a Tree Planted</u>, I said to myself gleefully.

We found Hendrix Lake surrounded by nearly bare hills on three sides. Wind blew through this gateway, across the desolate water. Snow patched the highest slopes.

We slowly turned into the lake's entrance, passing a former general store whose roof had caved in. Abandoned buildings clumped together in silence—old barracks made of gray cement blocks, a cafe with a faded sign, a row of empty offices. The main road, which paralleled the lakeshore, was lined by small houses, nearly all boarded up. A few had open windows through which we could see sofas and tables but no dishes or T.V.s or table lamps.

Three houses were still occupied—one had matching pink tricycles in the front yard. The back yard was enclosed by a tall, galvanized metal fence (to keep out the grizzlies). As we passed the children's house, a man wearing glasses watched us from the living room window.

I drove to an abandoned tennis court, where the road ended, and pulled up near the water. Across the lake, pine trees crowded the shoreline. A small, spruce-covered island rose to our left, toward the part of the lake that curved around where we could not see. The wind formed little breakers in the lake's center.

As soon as we got out of the car, a swarm of mosquitoes descended on us. Even with the wind blowing, the bugs hunted us.

With Jonathan in the stroller and Jessica on the basket behind, I took pictures of the lake and the abandoned houses. The last shot I reserved for Kristen kneeling by the stroller and handing Jonathan his bottle. The gray light from a cloudy sky illumined her gold hair and Jonathan's yellow curls. Jessica peeked her face around the stroller's neon-yellow frame, her auburn hair crowning her eyebrows and pink birthmark as she grinned widely. Different shades of blue gleamed from each child's eyes. The shutter clicked, the film rewound, and I set the camera down.

"Let's go this way," I pointed north of the cracked tennis court whose net fluttered, broken in the wind. This was the wildest path, away from the houses.

"I don't know..." Kristen hesitated.

"Ah, come on; it's daylight," I replied.

We walked hesitantly down a dirt path bordered by tall bushes. I could feel hidden eyes staring at us.

At a bend in the path, a calf's leg lay on the ground, cleanly severed. Kristen pointed at it. We stopped and stared at the object.

"Maybe we'd better walk on the main road, by the houses," I suggested.

"Weird," Kristen commented as we turned abruptly away. "Do you think there's a Satanic cult out here that sacrifices animals?"

I laughed, thinking we'd both lived too long in California.

"No, I think a cougar or a bear got ahold of that calf."

"Oh," Kristen commented, walking faster.

We strolled briskly by the empty houses and the house where someone still watched us through glass.

"Weird," Kristen said again as we stopped in front of the caved-in general store.

"Do you want to go up that hill to those other buildings?" I asked, pointing to the south end of the lake. "See, there are a couple of cars."

"Not really," Kristen replied. "This place is weird."

"I know what you mean. Let's go back to the lodge."

We hurried to the car and drove back down the rutted road. Only when we got back to the lodge did I realize that I had left the camera on the car's roof. It fell off somewhere between the lake and the lodge. All my beautiful pictures of trees and children were gone forever.

Maybe a grizzly bear found it.

I can only describe those images with words, like the Canadian flag, red and white in the shape of a maple leaf, blowing on its pole near the lodge.

A year later, Kristen and I went to another lake—in our local California mountains:

"That New World"

Outside, the misty air smells like snow. I'd love to see the snow fall, flakes on the children's cheeks and lashes...

We're driving toward a mountain lake. Both of the little ones are asleep, so Kristen and I park at the farthest shore of the lake and get out. We walk a few steps down to the water's edge. A lone fisherman sees us and moves around the bend, out of sight.

Mountains, patchworked with snow and pine trees, rise all around us. The sky grows darker, clouds heavy with snow. Grey waves lap at our feet, and I think of Hendrix Lake that we visited not so long ago.

"I'd like to tell you something profound that will change your life," I say. "But I'm not sure I can think of anything except this:

"Remember, all that we see now will pass away. Someday we will stand on the shores of a new world, eternal, where God will wipe all tears from our eyes."

My throat chokes up, and I can't speak for a moment.

"This last year has been hard for me, Kristen—the miscarriages and seeing people I know die of cancer. I've come too close to death; it's changed me."

I pause again and feel the wind sweep over the lake, cold. Kristen shivers beside me.

"Anyway, we're only here for awhile—strangers passing through. Don't get too caught up in this world. I don't mean the natural world, like this lake, but the secular, materialistic society which surrounds us. I made my worst mistakes when I got too engulfed in this world and forgot about Christ and His kingdom."

Kristen nods.

"When we meet in that new world, I hope we recognize each other," I add.

"Of course we will," she answers softly.

I think she's right, and for a second or two the rocks and water at our feet melt away, and a city surrounds us instead of mountains. A sea of glass leads to walls higher than we can see, made of precious stones like amethyst and emerald and sapphire. Light from the Lamb Himself shines from inside the city, through the rainbow walls, downward to us. Instead of clouds a new universe spreads above us, stars with no darkness between them, space with no distance or time.

Angels and beings covered with eyes and wings inhabit that city, and those who have suffered in this life wear robes washed white in the blood of the Lamb. They walk by the Tree of Life and drink from the stream that runs forever between its roots.

And the leaves of that Tree heal the nations.

"Well, I guess we'd better get back," I say, turning toward Kristen, whose arms cross over her chest, trying to hold out the biting mountain wind.

Ryan got into his share of trouble, too, when he was a teenager:

"Smoking at School"

Ryan was caught smoking in the boys' room at high school (my own son!). After school, I pick him up and give him a tour of Dr. Schinke's office.

"This is where they put x-rays of people's lungs. See that spot there? It's cancer. These three triangles warn you of the radiation room. Did you know that my friend Lori had both chemo and radiation? Radiation can cause the surface of your skin to burn black.

"This is The Chemo Room. See those three patients hooked up to I.V.s? It takes about two hours for the chemicals to go down from those plastic bags, through those plastic tubes, past the needle, and into your arm. Those white shawls keep you warm because the chemo feels cold as it enters your bloodstream. The nurses who mix the chemicals have to wear a mask, special smock, and gloves because the chemicals are so strong that <u>they</u> can cause cancer. Those plastic bowls are for when you get nauseated and throw up.

"This is the wig stand. This thing here measures your head to see what size you'll need. This box of Kleenex is for your family members who are afraid of losing you—and for you when you feel sorry for yourself or become terrified that you'll die. The Sparkletts cooler and these paper cups can give you water to ease your mouth sores after chemo treatments.

"Look, here is an eighteen-gauge needle. You'll get used to needles because you'll get daily shots and weekly blood draws.

"Any questions?"

Ryan was a lost soul, as in the day we talked about his future career possibilities:

"Eyes Like Seawater"

On one of Ryan's few days off, I drive him to a special "Mom and Me" lunch at Coco's restaurant (a friend is watching the little ones). Ryan sits next to me in the car and asks, "Are you proud of me?"

The other night, while Edd and I were talking to him after he got off work, late, he said, "I was an accident, wasn't I?" (referring to the circumstances of his birth).

"No, of course not; God made you," I replied.

Now, as we drive toward Coco's, I search for words to assure him, to improve his self-esteem. What can I give?

He's tall and awkward, like his father. His voice is always

loud (he was born without a volume control button). His light, freckled skin has turned dark, peeling from the sun in several layers. His hair is shaved close to his scalp. I touch the back of his neck and wonder what happened to the baby he was—or the little boy with the cowlick in his curly brown hair who stared intently at me once when we lived in Yorkshire and stated,

"You and dad don't treat me right."

True—he's easy to nag. He bumps into things, spills things, gets on people's nerves. An image of him at age nine pops into my mind—he stands in the doorway over a spilled salad bowl, grins, and says,

"Sorry, Mom."

His dad insisted that Ryan take Ritalin for years after Ryan's teachers complained that he couldn't sit still in the classroom. Did that drug help? Was there really something wrong with an active, outdoors boy stuck at a desk beneath fluorescent lights for six hours a day?

Our society is too quick to place labels on people: ADD, ADHD, Learning Disabled...

He can sit at a computer for hours, surfing the Net or playing games. He works hard at what interests him.

"Of course I'm proud of you," I say as I turn left into Coco's parking lot. "You've worked hard this summer. I think it's great that you want to be a beach lifeguard and a paramedic. You're suited to work outside, helping people."

Yes, Ryan has a good heart, a sweet heart, an innocent heart in many ways...He helps friends out to the point of being taken advantage of. He has a clever way with words, making people laugh at his stories that he illustrates with constantly moving hands.

Ryan listens to my praise, but I'm not sure he's convinced.

He came into the world when Kristen was still a baby. I was young and selfish and not quite ready for two children under two years old. Yet Ryan became my "cuddle bear." He'd let me hug him and kiss his nose while Kristen seemed content to play alone with her toys.

"Yeah, being a lifeguard and paramedic, you don't need to

be real smart," Ryan tells me as I park the car. He steps out into the sunlight and grins, his eyes like seawater.

※

Now Ryan's living in San Diego with his dad and stepmom. He's working hard as an auto mechanic (he always was good at putting things back together—like the pocket watch he disassembled when he was eight). Like me, he's not good at making money or managing it. He takes me to places like Book Expo America in Los Angeles, driving me in his new white Saturn that fits in well with the L.A. crowd. He helps me carry bags of books as we try to promote them to buyers. He tells me jokes and smiles a lot, and I say,

"You'd make a good youth pastor."

He laughs, and I wonder if he believes me.

When we return from our day trip to L.A., he plugs in his cell phone and places his car keys on the table.

"You're traveling light," I remark, wishing my life were less complicated.

He grins and gives the kids presents he cannot afford. He hugs me, tall and long-limbed, like a friendly bear. Then he sits on the floor in front of the T.V. and plays video games with Jessica and Jonathan, his sweet, loud laugh filling the room.

Nineteen

Eye of the Storm

I still have pain in my feet—but I'm sure it cannot compare to my neighbor Sherryl's:

"Helping Hands"

Our church recently joined another mountain church in a program called "Helping Hands." It is supposed to help single moms, senior citizens, and people with low income or disabilities. Sherryl, whose six-year-old daughter Sarah skates at the rink with Jessica and Jonathan, had to take an early retirement from the police department because some guy threw her against a wall and broke her neck. Sherryl's neck is better, but she still has a metal rod in it and gets searing migraines.

Sherryl has had six miscarriages—one more than I have. Most of the time, her now-ex-husband wasn't even there with her when she had her D&Cs. Sarah was her last pregnancy, so Sherryl ended with success.

But now Sherryl's ex-husband is constantly harassing her by taking her to court and scrutinizing any income she makes. She barely makes enough money to live on, and he makes $100,000 a year. She sacrifices to let Sarah skate at the rink part-time, giving her plucky little girl with the long blonde ponytail a chance to pursue a dream.

Sherryl needs lots of repairs around her house, and

sometimes she just needs a man to move stuff for her. I think she qualifies for "Helping Hands."

When I called the church who heads up the program, I spoke with their secretary. Now, church secretaries can be formidable people, and Jan was no exception.

"I'd like to recommend a friend of mine for the Helping Hands program," I started to explain. "She's a single mom and needs help around her house."

"Our church usually screens people before we put them on our list," she promptly replied. "Besides, I don't know who you are."

"I'm Lonna Williams, a local writer and member of another church on the mountain—the one who is partnering with you to do the Helping Hands program," I told her. "I'm just recommending a friend of mine who needs help."

"We usually have applicants screened before considering them," she repeated. "You have no idea how much we get taken advantage of. We've got to be careful."

I thought about that for a moment. We may live on a mountain, but families still break apart, people abuse drugs and children, there is poverty and sorrow...I looked out my bay window at the new leaves of spring and realized that even in this beautiful forest, there is trouble. And a lot of it is caused by our own foolish choices. Why do we always blame God?

"Well, my church secretary told me to call you," I explained, losing my patience. "You're not being very helpful. I just want to give you the name and phone number of my friend."

"I still don't know who you are," she responded. I imagined her dressed in a drill sergeant's uniform, complete with dark sunglasses and olive green hat.

"I'm Lonna Williams," I repeated. "You can get my books at the local bookstore, and I've been in the paper a few times. Check out my website. It's lonnawilliams.com. You can read all about me there. Or maybe you could call the pastor of my church or have my church secretary send a letter to you, proving that I really am a church member and not some stranger off the street. But I shouldn't have to explain all this to you. You should be more accommodating. After all, you call your program 'Helping Hands.' People who really need help would certainly be put off by your attitude!"

"I don't know who you are," she said a third time. "But you could try calling this number."

I thanked her (a little sarcastically) and wrote down the name and phone number she gave me. I dialed it several times, only to hear it ring and ring.

"I don't have time for this!" I announced out loud as Jessie and Jonathan played in the living room. "She gave me the home phone of some guy who doesn't have an answering machine!"

I thought, This isn't right.

And then I realized how angry things like this get me. I hate injustice. I can't stand it when people are pushed aside by an organization or a bully or a snippy church secretary. She should have been more helpful. Christians are <u>called</u> to risk being taken advantage of. Jesus said "Give to him who asks you, and from him who wants to borrow from you do not turn away." (Matthew 6:42). He didn't say "Be sure to screen him first." When Jesus fed the 5,000, a lot of people showed up just for the free food. A lot of people He healed ran joyfully off and never came back to thank Him. Did He turn anyone away?

Aren't we supposed to follow in Christ's steps?

I called Jan back.

"It's Lonna Williams again," I announced. "That person you don't know. But it's not important who I am. The important thing is that there's a woman in need, and we should help her. We Christians are supposed to be <u>servants</u>, just as Christ came not to be served but to serve. I called that phone number you gave me, and nobody answered."

"O.K. I'll call your church secretary, verify who you are, and pass your friend's name on to the man who heads up Helping Hands," she replied.

After I hung up, still exasperated over how long this was taking, I started mentally drafting the letter I was going to send to Jan's boss (the pastor of her church).

Sherryl told me that she tried going to that church, but when she shared her needs for firewood or sink repair, she was told "we'll pray for you."

I'm sure Sherryl could use a few prayers, as we all can. But it can't stop there. What good are mere words when <u>action</u> is needed? James hit this nail on the head when he wrote:

> "If a brother or sister is naked
> and destitute of daily food,
> And one of you says to them,
> "Depart in peace, be warmed and filled,"
> But you do not give them the things
> which are needed for the body,
> what does it profit?
>
> Thus also faith by itself,
> if it does not have works,
> is dead." (James 2:15 -17)

No wonder Christians sometimes get a bad reputation.

So I invited Sherryl over to my house. Little Sarah was more than happy to play, and Sherryl and I sat at my dining table and talked. She started giving me hints on how to make money on e-Bay (I've got to make money somewhere, and so far my books aren't doing that much on amazon.com). We walked into my computer room where I had amassed stuff that I wanted to take photos of and sell, when Sherryl burst into tears.

"Life has been so hard lately," she said between sobs. "Just as soon as I get over one battle, I'm hit with another. My family doesn't help me. My brother, who lives in the valley, has a ten-car garage in a million-dollar house. You should see the cars he puts in that garage. When I tell him I don't have enough money for food at the end of the month, he says that all his assets are tied up."

That really made me mad. "Your brother will pay for not helping you," I assure her. "We are supposed to help one another. You're either part of the solution or part of the problem. Jesus told His disciples that if they helped 'the least of these,' they helped Him. In the Final Judgment, Christ will divide the nations into two parts—those who helped, and those who didn't."

I realized I was ranting on, and Sherryl was not the one I was aiming my words at. I paused, thinking of my brother-in-law whose landlord still calls us once a week to report on what my brother-in-law is <u>not</u> doing.

"Yeah," Sherryl continued, interrupting my thoughts. "But that fact doesn't help me much. My phone was just disconnected because I owe money on my DSL Internet account that never even worked right. I can't list stuff on e-Bay!"

That fact hit me more than her brother's selfishness. I knew that having her phone disconnected was <u>not right</u>. She's a single mom who lives in the mountains where the roads get closed because of bad weather. She needs her phone!

"I'll call the phone company for you and try to get it reconnected," I suggested.

Sherryl stopped crying. We relocated back to my dining table where, using my remote headset phone, I called the phone company. After going through their menu, being put on hold, and talking to several different people, I got her phone reconnected.

"We got them to see the absolute truth that it isn't right to disconnect your phone because you owe a disputed Internet fee!" I exclaimed joyously. "In a battle like this, you need to find the right angle—the one argument that your opponent cannot, on moral grounds, refute."

Sherryl stared at me since I was sounding like an English professor lecturing on the process of logical argument.

"I actually did something concrete to help you!" I continued, clasping my hands together, delighted. "I justified my existence for today!"

"Well, thanks," Sherryl replied, heading for the door. "Now I'll be able to get back on e-Bay tonight."

She paused at the top of my thirty-six stairs and said,

"You know, when I read your book <u>Crossing the Chemo Room</u>, I felt like I was reading about my own life."

"Thanks," I replied, "that is why I write."

I watched her climb down my stairs and realized that she had just given me a greater gift than a telephone.

My church ended up helping her pay a few bills and then sent twelve men to move her shed and repair things around her house. We did this without the help of Jan's church.

―

"Strong Girls of the Bible"

Well, what can I say? Though I am a woman, I am also a fighter. Being a woman has its drawbacks in the public arena. Men in leadership positions have considered me illogical and emotional—even though I have a Master's degree, have been certified by the State of California to teach college English, and can lecture on logical argument.

The Bible gives examples of strong women. Rahab was a brave harlot who let the spies of Israel into the walled city of Jericho. Deborah was a Judge of Israel and a general of their army. She wrote the famous "Song of Deborah." Ruth left her own country and followed her step-mother to Israel. Ruth bravely reached out to the rich landowner Boaz who became her second husband. Ruth was great-grandmother of King David. Hannah went to the temple by herself and prayed for a son who became the prophet Samuel. The first Christian in Greece was a powerful merchant woman named Lydia, who opened her home to the apostle Paul.

I didn't fight cancer for nothing. You don't mess with a cancer survivor. We are warriors. We have learned, like Ripley in the movie <u>Aliens</u> or Selah in my own fantasy novels, that you can't run away from the monster. You've got to turn and face it. As I wrote in my journal:

"English Knight"

I wander into the bedroom alone and dress up for the Renaissance Faire. I put on my blue, puffy-sleeved blouse, black velvet bodice, and full skirt. I place a flower garland on my head, its pink ribbons trailing down my back. My blonde, wavy hair reaches past my shoulders. A silver Celtic cross and earrings finish the look.

I stare in the mirror and remember a time, not so long ago, when my reflection stared back, all pale and hairless, with dark circles beneath my eyes.

Now I look much better. I imagine another image in the mirror, a memory of England. In Ripon Cathedral, North Yorkshire, I once saw a statue of Saint George battling the dragon. In hues of silver and gold, the knight held a shield with a red cross on it and stuck the giant worm with his lance. The dragon writhed in agony beneath Saint George's triumphant feet.

I instinctively touch my chest to feel for lumps but find none. I had only one breast lump, deep inside where it could not be seen. I might have had lumps all over my body like Grandma Ruth did.

"You look like an Irish princess," Edd observes as he walks up behind me. He places his big hand on the nape of my neck.

"Thanks," I reply, imagining Edd in a knight's costume complete with metal armor and broadsword. He'd wear a green plaid Scottish sash to complement his reddish beard.

"I feel more like an English knight than an Irish princess, though," I admit.

Edd grins and kisses my hand. He bows, and in a broad English accent, says,

"Aye, m'lady, let me fetch ye the sword and shield."

And I thankfully reply:

"God has healed me, and I am still here, clothed in armor, ready to fight."

"Eye of the Storm"

Once I drove down the mountains in stormy weather. My friend Mary Hughes came with me, and when we had finished our shopping, we turned back. The mountains rose before us: ten thousand feet of rock covered by thick clouds. Lightning flashed as wind blew down, and the sound of thunder filled our ears.

"It's like driving toward the eye of the storm," Mary said in a hushed voice.

"Yes," I replied. "Isn't it wonderful?"

Twenty

Technology

My life has been shaped by technology. I was born for the computer age. I have benefited from electricity, cell phones, the Internet, and advances in medicine. Yet technology has its harmful side. You don't have to look far to realize this: radioactive waste, landfills brimming with plastic, nuclear bombs, air pollution from cars and factories, toxic chemicals, global warming...We take the bad with the good.

Technology caused my cancer, cured it, and left me with side effects. Even now, I'm afraid to get medical tests:

"Getting My Breast Tests"

I finally broke down and got my yearly breast tests. I don't like check-ups anymore—not since I had cancer. It's been six years since my treatment, but terror still lurks in the back of my mind: what if they find something?

I show up at our little mountain hospital's radiology department and endure over an hour of modern torture. The mammogram technician, who has been doing this for 30 years, makes me stand in awkward positions next to a big white machine with railings and rectangular edges. As she squashes my left breast in the cold, metal x-ray tray, I feel like I'm making love to a robot.

"Ignorance is not bliss," she tells me brightly. "It's better to find something before it gets too big to treat," she adds before stepping behind the x-ray shield.

Yeah, I know, I think as she tells me to hold my breath. I remember the CAT-scan tube where I had to hold my breath every few seconds as x-rays swirled around my body and red laser lights blinked on and off. My head feels light, my heart starts beating faster, and I try not to have another anxiety attack.

"I probably got cancer because of all the chest x-rays I had as a child," I tell the technician when she comes out from behind the shield and helps pose my other breast against the machine. "I had bronchitis a lot. Those old x-ray machines put out a lot more radiation, didn't they?"

The technician stares at me for a moment. She has sensible short, curly hair and a green smock.

"I won't contradict you," she finally says. "I could tell you some things about radiology 30 years ago. But now, this mammogram machine puts out as much radiation as you get by stepping out into the sunlight."

"And staying in the sun all day?"

"No, just stepping out into it."

I hope she's right.

Next, the technician takes me to a dark room. I lie down on a hospital bed next to a boxy tan ultrasound machine. She puts liquid on the soundmaker pad and passes it slowly across each breast. I glance at the screen—black with wispy white shapes like clouds.

I close my eyes, breathe deeply, and let my mind drift away from the small dark hospital room.

I imagine that cathedral in England again. At the foot of an ornate altar, I look up at a gilded statue of Saint George. In one hand, he holds a shield with a red cross on it. With the other hand he thrusts a lance into a writhing red dragon.

I imagine a dragon sleeping in my right breast, next to the scar made five years ago. Will the passing of the ultrasound pad awaken it?

No, no—it's gone now, I assure myself. God really did let

me survive. These tests, though terrifying as facing a fifty-foot dragon, are for my good. They show the hidden things inside.

I try to read the technician's facial expressions.

"Do you see anything unusual?" I ask, peeking at the cryptic white shapes on the screen.

"I don't read the results," she reminds me. "But maybe you can catch the radiologist before he leaves. If I hurry these films to him, he'll read them for you."

She sets the pad next to the machine, and I get dressed, praying I won't have to wait for the test results.

The radiologist waits for me. He shakes my hand—a small, Asian man with glasses. He points to the films like x-rays on his backlit wall.

"Nothing to worry about," he says with an accent. "Only one small cyst in each breast."

"Thank you," I say, unable to tell where those cysts are by looking at the white and black images. I go home. I'm having friends over tonight for my son's seventh birthday party. He was a baby when I found that lump in my breast.

"I don't want any radiation in <u>my</u> breast," my friend Cherie says as she sits at my kitchen table. "I've never had a mammogram."

"I have," Mary Pat states. "I've had lots of tests."

Several children run past us, playing hide and seek.

"Get it done, Cherie," I suggest. "There's not much radiation in a mammogram. It's better to know than not, even though the test may scare you. You wouldn't want to be told that you have advanced breast cancer and six months left to live, especially since you have four young children."

Cherie stares at me, thinking about my words. "Are you sure there's not much radiation in a mammogram?" she asks.

"It's like walking outside in the sunlight," I reply.

"Bill Gates and Paul"

Speaking of technology, I'd like to contrast two famous people: Bill Gates of Microsoft and the Apostle Paul.

Bill Gates is an icon of the late Twentieth Century. In 1995, Time magazine put Bill Gates on its cover. Gates' glasses reflected light as he held a bolt of glowing electricity between his thumb and forefinger.

"Master of the Universe" the caption read.

In 1997, Time put another photo of Bill Gates on their cover. The new article gave more insight into Gate's personality and past (I've added some additional information collected since then).

Gates was fiercely rebellious as a child, yelling to get his way, stuck to his futurevision like a compass needle northward. He stole the idea of Windows from his rival Steve Jobs, founder of Macintosh Computers, then formed a monopoly on Internet and computer software.

He would like to create a silicon-based creature to rival us carbon-based ones.

When the Time interviewer asked Gates if he believed in the human soul, Gates replied, as he sat in a fancy restaurant,

"I have no evidence of that."

He rocked back and forth in his seat, his arms over his abdomen, repeating,

"I have no evidence of that."

Gates is one of the richest men in the world. He married a woman who worked for Microsoft. They have two children. His Megahouse is fully automated with a computer in every room and cameras watching all the guests. He has written books about the future of computers and the Internet. And he's had problems in anti-trust courts.

Now let's look at Paul of Tarsus.

Paul was born in the First Century. He was originally named Saul. He was both a Roman citizen and a Jew who studied under the great teachers of the Law and zealously opposed Christians, even to their death. When a crowd stoned the disciple Stephen in Jerusalem, Saul guarded their cloaks, consenting to their act. He pursued Christians, a sort of First Century Bounty Hunter.

Then he met Christ on the road to Damascus.

Not everyone gets blinded by the light. Saul fell from his horse as he heard a Voice,

"Saul, Saul, why are you persecuting me?"

Saul replied, "Who are you, Lord?"

"I am Jesus, whom you are persecuting...Arise and go into the city, and you will be told what you must do."

So Saul was led to a friend's house where he waited for a humble man named Ananias to come and pray for him. Ananias was reluctant when asked to help the notorious Bounty Hunter. But the Lord said,

"Go, for he is a chosen vessel of Mine to bear My name before Gentiles, kings, and the children of Israel. For I will show him how many things he must suffer for My name's sake."

Ananias obeyed, and Saul was transformed. He regained his sight and changed his name to Paul (ironic, since "Saul" was the name of the first King of Israel, a tall and noble man—and "Paul" meant "small"). Paul spread the gospel to the Mediterranean world, which was perfect for traveling thanks to the Roman Empire's tight control and well-built roads. He worked with his own hands as a tentmaker, refusing to live off the donations of the churches he helped establish. He was beaten, hungry, poorly clothed, homeless, stoned, shipwrecked, imprisoned. He was probably a widower with no biological children. He walked on his own sandaled feet, speaking the Good News to Jews and Gentiles, women and men, slaves and Kings.

His last letter was to Timothy, his "beloved son in the faith." The year was A.D. 60. Paul was old, tired, and chained in Rome for the last time—not under house arrest but in a criminal prison.

As he wrote, he probably sat at a wood table near an oil lamp. He was most likely an ordinary-looking man, with weak eyes and a speech impediment. He must have worn rags, unwashed, trying to steady his shivering hand as he penned,

"Remember that Jesus Christ, of the seed of David,
was raised from the dead according to my gospel,
for which I suffer trouble as an evildoer,
even to the point of chains;
but the word of God is not chained."

He might have paused and stared up at the dripping stone walls.

"For I am already being poured out as a drink offering,
and the time of my departure is at hand.
I have fought the good fight,
I have finished the race,
I have kept the faith.
Finally, there is laid up for me the crown
of righteousness, which the Lord,
the righteous judge, will give to me
on that Day, and not to me only but also
to all who have loved His appearing."

Paul glimpsed that future city, that New Jerusalem adorned like a bride for her husband. Yet he also saw the rat in the corner, the filthy straw at his chained feet, the cracked clay pot of unclean water on the table. He pulled his tunic closer over his shoulders and wrote:

"Bring the cloak that I left with Carpus at Troas
when you come—and the books,
especially the parchments...
Do your best to come before winter."

Contrast this image of Paul with Bill Gates who sat at the restaurant table and said he had no evidence for the human soul. Paul understood Gates' position. Before he was imprisoned, Paul wrote:

"But the natural man does not receive
the things of the Spirit of God,

for they are foolishness to him;
nor can he know them,
because they are spiritually discerned...

Let no one deceive himself. If anyone
among you seems to be wise in this age,
let him become a fool that he may become wise.
For the wisdom of this world is foolishness
with God, for it is written,
'He catches the wise in their own craftiness.'" (1 Corinthians 2:14 and 3:18-19)

Bill Gates and the Apostle Paul—two men of stubbornness, purpose, and vision—separated by centuries of time and material and spiritual worlds.

Yet I am grateful for both of them. I pick up my Bible and head for my computer room, thankful to Paul for his inspirational letters and to Bill Gates for Microsoft Word. I smile, considering thesis, antithesis, and synthesis as I type black letters on the glowing white screen.

Tonight I will dream of technology, of Bill Gates and his Empire. I will see Microsoft Corporation as a kind of 3D temple on the Internet—a huge structure with sold block walls and geometric shapes, with stone floors and passages I can explore by the click of a mouse. Microsoft Corp. will compete with Solomon's Temple for size and glory—but without the glowing cloud of God's presence. Then, in my dream, New Jerusalem will rise out of the west—in colors brighter than clouds painted by the sun, in dimensions greater than even Bill Gates or the Internet can create.

Twenty-One

The Josefina Doll

Have you ever had a gift rejected? It feels like a slap in the face, doesn't it? This happened to Jessica recently. All on her own she decided to use the allowance she had saved up for several months to buy her best friend a special doll so that they could play together. The girl's parents decided the gift was too extravagant (and that we probably expected it to be repaid somehow), so they brought the doll back to our house, all wrapped up in its box like a coffin. As they explained all the logical, sound psychological reasons for returning the gift, I walked alone into the kitchen. I didn't want to see Jessica cry. The gift was precious, given freely. I knew its rejection brought Jessie pain.

Does God feel that way when we reject His love?

Then I heard that the dad had called the story into the popular pop-psychology radio show of Dr. Laura. I tried calling Dr. Laura's 800 number. After waiting for an hour of busy signals, someone finally answered.

"What is your question?" she asked in an impatient voice.

I started telling the Josefina Doll story, and she interrupted me.

"You have to have a question."

I tried to ask one, but she hung up on me. I stared, amazed, at the buzzing phone.

So I decided to do the logical thing—write Dr. Laura a letter:

May 17, 2002
Dear Dr. Laura,

It truly is a small world we live in. I am from a mountain town, and I hardly ever listen to the radio. I'm too busy with my children and promoting my published books (you can check out my science fiction, fantasy, and cancer survival stories on amazon.com or my website). But two days ago (Wednesday, May 15) a friend of mine called into your radio program and told my daughter's story of The Value of a Gift. I would never even have known this if another friend hadn't heard that program and called to tell me.

My daughter Jessica is in the American Girls' Club. This group of elementary-aged girls meet semiweekly to study history in a fun way, via the American Girls curriculum which features dolls that come complete with books about their time in history, period costumes, and accessories. For a year and a half Jessica (who gets the American Girl catalog) had been bugging me to get her the "Kirstin" doll (a plucky blonde who emigrated with her family from Sweden to the American prairie in 1854). Her doll finally arrived two weeks ago. Then, she got the brilliant idea that she would buy her best friend a Josefina doll (a Mexican beauty who lived in 1824). That way, the two girls could play dolls together.

This week, she gave the doll to her friend. Her parents objected, saying the gift was too expensive, and the doll was returned to a confused and crying Jessica.

True, the doll cost about $130.00 (including shipping). But Jessica earned that with her allowance that she had been saving up for months. She worked especially hard since January when I broke my ankle and had to wear a cast for two months in a three-storey mountain house. Financial advisors often suggest that, if possible, a child should be paid a weekly allowance equal to her age. Thus, you can see how Jessica could have saved $130.

Jessie meant the doll as a gift. Freely given. No strings attached. She is not the type of girl to hold the gift over the friend's head like a debt to be repaid. She wanted to do something wonderful and surprising and generous for her best friend.

My question is, have we as Americans lost The Value of a Gift? Have we become so self-sufficient and rewards-oriented that we miss the point of receiving something we do not need to repay?

I am reminded of the Christian idea of grace—that God's own Son came to live among us, die, and rise again to give us eternal life. The Apostle Paul exclaimed, "Thanks be to God for His indescribable gift" (2 Corinthians 9:15). If one is not a Christian but believes in some sort of God, surely one can also see that the very gift of life and of the natural world around us (the part we haven't spoiled, anyway) is something we could never hope to repay—no matter how hard we worked.

I think the friend's father missed the value of Jessica's gift. I know that he is a psychologist in a public school, and that he was taking into consideration appropriate boundaries. But why must a price tag be put on a gift, anyway? Why is it OK to give something that costs $15 but not something that costs $130? If the parents had not known how much the doll cost, would they have allowed their daughter to keep it? Shouldn't one consider the source of the gift and the motives? If Jessica were a teenage boy trying to win over a teenage girl with bribes, the case would be different.

I have a Master's degree in English and used to teach college before deciding to stay home with Jessica and her little brother. I taught logical argument, research, and literature. There is a short story by American writer O. Henry called "The Gift of the Magi." Set in the early Twentieth Century, it is about a newlywed couple who have no money for their first Christmas together. The wife has one asset: beautiful long hair. The husband has one valuable heirloom: a gold watch handed down from his father. The wife decides to cut off her hair and sell it in order to buy a chain for her husband's watch. The husband decides to sell his watch in order to buy a lovely comb for his wife's hair.

They are both surprised on Christmas morning, moved beyond words at the generosity and self-sacrifice represented in their gifts.

Maybe we could take a lesson from Christianity, nature, or O. Henry. Maybe we shouldn't refuse a gift that is given freely, from the heart.

I wish you would tell this other side of the story you aired on May 15. Thanks for taking time to read this.

Lonna Lisa Williams

I put a copy of Dr. Laura's letter into Josefina's box and mailed her back. A few weeks later, I received a letter from the American Girl Customer Service worker who was touched by Jessica's story:

"Jessica shows the qualities that we at American Girl try to promote. She must be a special girl to have given such a gift."

A few more weeks passed, and I didn't hear back from Dr. Laura. I decided to write her another letter:

June 20, 2002
Dear Dr. Laura,
I FAXed the enclosed letter to you on May 17 but heard nothing back, so I thought I'd write you with an update.

I received a letter from American Girl, and I'm enclosing a copy. Also, I'm enclosing an inspirational little story about a man who gave away money at a mall (because it relates to my idea of The Value of a Gift).

My daughter Jessica is still hurt that her gift was returned, and her doll Kirsten still does not have another American Girl doll to play with. Jessica's friend's mother told the Josefina doll story to the other mothers at the American Girls' Club, and they pretty much agreed that the gift was inappropriate. I was not there to add my contrasting opinion.

The mother added that maybe it would be better if Jessica didn't play much with her daughter much anymore.

A gift that meant well has become a divisive issue. I think it is an issue worthy of more discussion on your radio program.

Thanks for your time,
Lonna Lisa Williams

I'm still waiting to hear from Dr. Laura.

I know what it feels like for a gift to be refused. I've sent many copies of my books to people or organizations who never even acknowledged receiving them—or who sent them back unopened. I've had my books rejected by some of the best publishers and literary agents in the world. And I personally hand-delivered one to Carrie Fisher:

"Searching for Carrie Fisher"

My local mountain newspaper advertised a Women in Business Expo in the valley. Carrie Fisher would be speaking. I had been wanting to meet her for years, ever since we were nineteen at the same time, and she made her debut as Princess Leia in <u>Star Wars</u>. As a young adult, I read <u>Postcards from the Edge</u> and enjoyed her sarcasm, sense of humor, and clever use of words (I even stole one of her lines). I kept up with her writing career, reading articles on the Internet and watching A&E Network's profile of her on <u>Biography</u>. But the biggest reason I wanted to meet Carrie was because she has lived a crazy life, too, though entirely different from mine.

So I got a babysitter for the kids and drove down the mountain to the valley heat and freeways. It took two hours one way, in traffic, to reach the Fairgrounds. After parking on the edge of the huge lot, I hiked to the Fairplex building where the convention was being held, clutching my briefcase with its precious cargo of one signed copy of <u>Crossing the Chemo Room</u>.

Four years ago Carrie Fisher was a keynote speaker at the Maui Writers' Conference. I was all set to go, reservations made, when we had to cancel the trip. I sent the first few chapters of my manuscript anyway, care of the hotel which hosted the conference. I never heard anything. If she got the typed, double-spaced pages, she probably threw them into the hotel trash bin (who would want to haul such a big manuscript all the way back to L.A.?). Last summer, before I finally went to the Maui Writers' Conference, I asked the conference staff to forward my book to Carrie. Eventually, I got the package back, undeliverable.

So I brought the same book to the valley, hoping to hand it to Carrie personally. When I finally found the conference headquarters, I wandered through the huge, barn-like building which was bigger than an ice rink. Its concrete floors were shiny and smooth, almost like ice, and I couldn't help but glide a few strokes on my slick-bottom shoes.

The conference workers told me that Carrie would be speaking during lunch, and the best time to hand her the book would be right after she finished. I found a seat near the front and waited, barely picking at my pasta salad. After awhile, someone pointed Carrie out to me. She was sitting at her table. Her hair was short, with blonde streaks. She wore dark-rimmed reading glasses and a short black dress over a figure that was not as thin as it had once been. She didn't look much like she did twenty-five years ago when she was Princess Leia. I don't look much like I did then, either.

Someone blasted the <u>Star Wars</u> theme over the loudspeaker as Carrie ascended stairs to the stage. A scene from the movie flashed through my mind, and for a moment I saw a slender, dark-haired young woman in a flowing white dress. Those famous braids wound around the sides of her head as she bent to insert a secret message into a droid. She paused and looked over her shoulder as an evil Empire hunted her down.

"If that music followed you around twenty-five years later," Carrie said, removing her glasses and touching the podium mic with one hand, "you'd be crazy too."

The audience laughed, and Carrie smiled—that impish, lopsided smile beneath sparkling brown eyes.

Your smile has not changed, I thought.

Carrie was referring to her bout with mental illness. She

nearly lost her mind once when she was stuck on a manic-depressive high. Now she is an advocate for people getting the medications they need for bipolar disorders.

Carrie's speech was funny, irreverent, and off-the-wall. Some people were probably offended, but I thought how honest she was being and how harsh her life has been (her father abandoned her when she was a baby, she got heavily into drugs, her daughter's father abandoned her for a man, and she didn't know how to deal with her intense mood swings). I listened and laughed and clapped at the appropriate times. She asked for questions but didn't call on me though I raised my hand high. Then I walked over toward her, with the rest of the women who wanted to meet her. They thronged around her, wanting autographs or photos.

I thought about other famous people I've met. I spoke to Leonard Nimoy briefly on a naval base, near a moored aircraft carrier where he had been directing and starring in <u>Star Trek IV</u>. He seemed a little annoyed when I asked for his autograph (which I promptly lost). I saw Prince Andrew of England from a distance once when he flew in on a helicopter to that same naval base. I chatted with C. Everett Coop, former Surgeon General for the United States, in a line at Heathrow airport in London.

Why does the public gravitate toward celebrities? Because we see them on T.V.? In Jesus' time, there was no mass media. Jesus never appeared on the Big Screen. People came to him in person, thronging around Him, longing for a word or a touch.

My thoughts faded as Carrie Fisher finally stepped toward me.

I am meant to be here, I wanted to say as I stood there with the book in my hand, God sent me to give you a gift.

But instead I remarked,

"My question is 'Do you ice skate?'"

She looked at me for a moment, surprised.

"My daughter does," she replied.

"Come up to the mountains," I invited. "And skate at the rink with us sometime."

I handed her the copy of <u>Crossing the Chemo Room</u> that held her name. It also contained my business card, a picture of my kids with Michelle Kwan, and a map to the mountains. She held the book for a moment and then passed it to her assistant.

"I did hard drugs too," I confided as the crowd pressed around us. "I had chemotherapy. I'm a cancer survivor."

"Oh," she said as the crowd moved her away.

Determined, I handed my camera to a man standing by.

"Take my picture with her, please," I requested.

Carrie was swept back toward me like driftwood on a wave, and I put my arm around her shoulder for a second as the photographer snapped the shot.

Carrie's assistant reminded her that they had to get back to L.A. before rush-hour traffic. I watched as she guided Carrie toward the side exit.

As I glided a little more over the slick concrete and thought about ice skating at the rink, I wondered what Carrie would do with my book. Would it end up in a forgotten pile of gifts the public had given her? Would it be tossed into a trash can—there to sit for awhile like hidden treasure until it was hauled to the dump?

Or would she read it?

Well, at least I have the photo to remember, I thought as I drove all the way home.

When I got the photo developed, I couldn't believe how awful I looked. It was the worst photo I had ever taken. I forgot to remove my glasses as I stood there, towering over Carrie, my blonde hair looking like I had just stuck my head out a car window, and my red face smiling so big that I looked like a mindless idiot. Carrie, who has much more experience on the receiving end of a camera, had taken her glasses off and tilted her head a little, wearing a small and ladylike smile as her hair perfectly framed her alabaster face.

Carrie will probably never remember me and the few words I exchanged with her. But if she reads my book, the long journey to give it to her will be worth everything.

I may never know what Carrie Fisher did with my gift. But that's the risk of giving, isn't it?

"Mariko's Gift"

Sometimes the giver needs to receive. Once I lent my <u>Crossing the Chemo Room</u> book to a woman at the ice rink. Her name is Mariko, and she is from Tokyo but now lives in Palm Springs. She drives her daughter Saki up the mountain five days a week, a one-hour drive each way. Mariko is shy and quiet, surprisingly tall, with short dark hair and glasses. She's always wearing slacks and running shoes. She smiled when she returned my book, handing me a flowered thank-you note and a box of Godiva chocolates.

I have hand-delivered or mailed dozens of my books, and very few people have sent me thank-you notes. I stared at Mariko's handwriting in blue ink in a fine and careful style. I felt surprised beyond measure as I read the simple words. Then I held up the gold-wrapped box of expensive chocolate. It was covered with a green bow that glittered like ice.

"Thanks, Mariko," I said, hugging her, tears clouding my eyes. It had been a long week filled with rejection letters and closed doors.

"I will always write for chocolate."

Twenty-Two

A Place Beyond Pain

Today I feel like throwing tomatoes. At what, I'm not sure. Or maybe I could drive to the far side of the mountain, climb to the highest peak of 12,000 feet, stand on top of a rock, and scream. Instead, I lock myself up in the outhouse at Jessica's horse camp and cry (I've got PMS). Outside the other parents are watching their children ride horses in the ring. One dad, who has a toddler at his feet, is taking videos of his daughter with her black velvet English riding hat and coat, sitting proudly in the saddle of a quarterhorse. He is a single parent whose wife recently left him. I cry for him. Why do marriages have to go wrong?

In the outhouse, I think of other reasons to cry.

This week, a local jeweler told me that he lost custody of his daughter who is Jonathan's age. He was so angry and hurt that he hit the wall hard with a hammer (he was remodeling his store at the time). I couldn't think of anything good to say until after I left the store, and it probably wouldn't have helped him much to know that he isn't the only one who has gone through such a thing.

After my divorce, when Ryan was only eight and Kristen ten, my ex-husband hired a "hardball" layer and got full physical custody of the children. I got dragged through the hell of Family Court. I could see my children only every other weekend, and for awhile not even then (add that to the guilt that the divorce was largely my idea). Then my ex-husband and his wife took

Kristen and Ryan with them to Washington State for two years, when I was going through chemotherapy and needed teenagers around to help me with a baby and a toddler and all the trauma of cancer.

Why do ex-spouses pursue revenge?

Another friend told me his oldest daughter is graduating from high school and going to college at the end of summer. He sounded heartbroken, and I thought of nothing to say. But later I thought,

At least she will still be in the same State, and you have her heart...

Why do children have to grow up?

Of course, I decided (in that smelly outhouse) to cry for myself too.

Why do babies have to die before they're born?

After five years of miscarriages, the whole reproductive thing makes me sick. When my friend Cherie (the one who had a stillborn boy) told me the "good news" that she was pregnant again, I got a horrible taste in my mouth like ashes. I've had to sit in church over these past few months and watch Cherie's belly grow to obnoxious proportions.

Pregnant women and women with newborns seem to be everywhere, reminding me...

Another woman just had her baby, and last Sunday she and her husband stood in front of the church door so that everyone could admire their firstborn son.

I went in the other door.

And inside the church I sat in the same row as a pregnant woman who looks older than I do, and I watched the big stained glass window with its cross—red and yellow against blue and green. The mountain sunlight shone through, and I could see the swallows behind the glass, flitting back and forth, making their nests...

It's an over-forty thing. Trying to have a baby over 40 is like playing Russian roulette—using a six-cylinder gun with five bullets in it. Those actresses who have babies at 45 usually get egg donors and then stay in bed the whole 9 months with servants to wait on them and the best doctors to check them all the time.

Pregnant women can be so smug. They are always smiling, with the "see what I can do" look on their faces. They're always introspective, rubbing their bellies, expecting everyone to oooh and aaah over them and open doors for them.

Every time I look at a pregnant woman, I feel like a hot iron is pressing against my bare skin. I feel like a mule with a carrot dangling in front of my face, on the end of a string, just out of reach. I feel like I was invited to a feast and then forced to sit in the shadows and watch everyone else dine on delicacies. So I came up with a list:

Lonna's Top Ten Things She Hates About Miscarriages

Number One—the <u>emotional torment</u>—feeling that the pregnant woman next to me at the bookstore is holding a sword to my heart when she really doesn't know who I am or why I'm staring at her belly.

Number Two—the <u>emotional torment</u>, part two. While looking for picture frames in a box, I open the empty silver frame with places for additional photos inside and discover the almost-forgotten sonogram photo of baby Michael, all white and fuzzy against the black background of my womb as he lay dying at fifteen weeks...four years ago.

Number Three—the <u>emotional torment</u>, part three. Waking up at three in the morning after yet another dream about holding a perfect newborn girl with all ten tiny fingers and toes. I stare at the dark ceiling, cry, and ask questions.

Number Four—the <u>questions</u>. Here they are: why, why, why, why, why?

Number Five—the <u>humiliation</u> of telling people I'm pregnant, daring to think that my announcement means I'll actually have a living, healthy baby in a few months, and then having to tell everybody that I won't. And, gee, I wasn't kidding. I really was pregnant. That little test with the two pink lines (and my body) told me. So what happened? If I don't understand it, how can I explain it to a six-year-old?

Number Six—the <u>physical torment</u> of gaining weight, getting nauseous, having contractions, and dealing with postpartum depression—all without a baby. Then continuing to live in a body that still produce hormones and eggs (with all the necessary PMS and migraines).

Number Seven—having to <u>learn to trust</u> God again (after all, didn't He promise to work everything out for good somehow?).

Number Eight—instead of getting flowers and tiny blue booties, I get sympathy cards.

Number Nine—having to <u>wait</u> to see the whole thing make sense (Maybe I will learn to be content with what I have, go into menopause, and figure that the whole baby idea was one of my most stupid ever. Or maybe I'll adopt a child from Russia. Or maybe I'll get pregnant one last time and actually have a baby...). So that leads me to:

Number Ten—not being able to give up <u>hope</u> but knowing that I don't have much chance of another healthy pregnancy.

I know these feelings are extremely immature and should be at the beginning of this book instead of near the end. By now, I should have come to a happy acceptance of my miscarriages and the "closure" everyone talks about in pop psychology. I never wanted to end up in my forties, bitter about not having another child, envious of those who are having one. But I can't help how I feel right now, and I don't particularly want someone to speak sensible words like "get over it."

I know women who are vegetarians and naturally thin though they don't particularly exercise. They eat mostly raw food—no meat, caffeine, wheat, or sugar (what is left?). Give me chocolate and tea! I say when I am having PMS. Forget dieting!

"Doesn't she look great?" other people say to me when a pregnant woman walks by, and I can't help but think that she isn't much younger than I am and doesn't look it.

Someone hung a "New Mother's Ministry" sign on the wall in the ladies' bathroom at church. It invites people to make a meal for a woman who has just had a baby. I want to rip it off the wall and tear it into little pieces. Or better yet, put a sign next to it that says "Grieving Mothers Ministry—bring a meal to a woman whose child is in the hospital or who has just had a miscarriage."

Why do people give so much attention to new mothers, whose world is already filled with the joy of a new life—and ignore mothers who have lost a child? People would rather go to a party than a wake. We don't know what to say when someone suffers. We don't want to deal with grief and loss. But why not throw a party for women who have miscarried? We could give them a safari hat, a backpack, a walking stick, and a map of exotic places...so they know that, whether or not they have another baby, they can get on with their life and explore.

Motherhood hurts. From the moment you conceive, you are in pain of one type or another. Then there's the labor and delivery (they don't call that "delivery" for nothing). Then there's the constant demand of a baby who keeps you up all night, then chasing around toddlers, then driving elementary-aged children from activity to activity.

A child is like an octopus: eight arms going in different directions, grasping things, collecting bright objects to put in its den, throwing up inkclouds of evasion...I tell Jessica that when I became a mother, I lost part of my brain. I constantly pick up white lint from our dark red carpet. I babysit animals and clean out cages. I wake up in the middle of the night to think about the long list of things I need to do the next day, then have trouble getting going in the morning, feeling like I'm on another Merry-go-Round, spinning in circles, getting nothing done...Jonathan runs everywhere he goes and chatters constantly. He annoys Jessica; Jessica bullies him.

Children don't appreciate your efforts, talk back, and drive you to tears.

In the long run, when both our stories are over, will Cherie be better off than I because she had another child? Someday all her children, like mine, will be grown and gone. A woman cannot continuously wrap her life around her children. A woman can do more than have babies.

We must learn that, for we will not always be able to have babies. Even when we are young, we can't count on getting pregnant—or pregnancies turning out right.

I know that I'm trying to rationalize my immaturity, envy, and bitterness. Well, if I could live in a "no pregnancy zone," maybe I really would "get over it."

I saw Nina recently (my Russian friend who found out she was pregnant at the same time I did last year). She was big with her twins, filling out her blue print dress like a blossom ready to burst into flower. She invited me to her baby shower. I avoided answering her. Nina seemed apologetic and not the least bit smug, as she spoke to me in her charming accent. But I still couldn't bring myself to her baby shower. It will probably take me six months after her twins are born to visit her. When I am in the grocery store, I can handle smiling and waving at a baby six months old or older. Just don't ask me to look at the newborns.

I gave away all of the baby clothes I saved from Jessica and Jonathan (except for a few keepsakes). I had been carting around all those extra bags for years, hoping to have another child. So when Sherryl said she could sell them on e-Bay, I just gave them to her. Later that night I woke up at 3:00 a.m. and told a surprised Edd,

"I gave away all those baby clothes! That means we will never have another child..."

I always dream in color. Sometimes I dream that I'm wandering along an Alaskan valley surrounded by snow-topped mountains. I see tall evergreen trees against the dark blue sky and a white-foamed river among red rocks. Other times, I dream about a tiny, perfect little baby girl with pink skin and a heart-shaped mouth. She's wrapped in a white blanket that glows with its own light. Crescent-shaped, she is cradled in my arms. I hold her and say,

"I'm sorry you didn't come to live with us. I saw you in the moon."

And then she fades away.

I think about the love Edd and I share—the love that brought us Jessica and Jonathan—and I wonder how something so beautiful could end in a miscarriage. I wish I had never been handed a miscarriage, that I had my tubes tied after Jonathan was born.

Like Frodo with the Ring of Doom, I wish that none of this had happened.

"You should focus not on what you've lost but on what you still have," is a line I heard in a late-night movie once when I couldn't sleep. I look at friends of mine who have several small children and think, I couldn't handle another child anyway. Wanting a baby must have been temporary insanity.

But seeing Jonathan playing with a toddler in front of the ice rink makes me sad.

"I want a little brother," he comes up and says to me.

I bend down and reply, "I don't know...I'm pretty busy with the two of you. Besides, it looks like you'll have to take that request up with God."

Jonathan stares at me for a moment, thinking. He finally states, "I could take care of him."

He goes back to stand among the tall wildflowers, picks up a dried dandelion, and blows seeds toward the baby. The wind catches the seeds, and for a moment they hang in the air, lit by the late afternoon sun as it slants through evergreen trees. They sparkle like gold chips or fairy dust, and then they are gone...

Jonathan will never have a baby brother. In the distance, a clock tolls the hour in long, mournful tones, and I realize that all babies must grow old.

And I know a
Place Beyond Pain
Deeper Than Tears
Without Words

And most of us have been there. And we have survived.

But, in the meantime, where do we put the pain?

We should be able to take the pain, lay it at the foot of the Cross, and leave it there.

Twenty-Three

Easter in the Mountains

I finally have a home. I, the fatherless "white trash" child who lived out of her car, who received hand-me-down clothes from churches, who knew trailer parks and temporary mansions and alcoholic relatives and cancer and miscarriages, have found the best place in the world. I searched a long time for it—all across America, in Germany and England, China, Canada, the Phillipines, and even Hawaii.

My little California mountain town by a lake cannot compare to any of the places I've visited. Only North Yorkshire, in England where my ancestors lived, is a close second. I could have stayed there in my Yorkshire village at my friend Carol's farmhouse—with Kristen and Ryan in the village school and free pony riding lessons and invitations to tea. I explored the open footpaths across moors, over rock walls, through sheep pens, farmers' fields, hills, and streams. I loved the history and architecture of centuries'-old manors, castles, and abbeys, the fairy tales and Knights of the Round Table and Shakespeare, the many colors of green in evergreen trees and grass. I had an English accent that could fool the English.

I cried all the way back to America.

But I'm glad I returned, met Edd, had Jessica and Jonathan, moved to the mountains.

In our little mountain town, we greet each other at the Post Office or the supermarket. We exchange items in the hardware store without a receipt and, instead of change back, get our pick of cookies or soda. We have homeschool groups that meet for Mom's Night Out or field trips. We send each other emails. We shovel snow together in winter and drive on twisty, foggy roads in spring. We share forest fires and drought. We are tied together with these mountains, islands of evergreen trees and ferns and rocks above the vast desert valleys.

I, like Selah, love the Summit, where vistas reach out in all directions—to sheer rock cliffs and heather-covered slopes and lakes and waterfalls—to the sandy valley below one side of the mountain and the millions of city lights below the other. From the Rim you can lie back and watch meteors streak across the sky or the eclipse of a full moon. The air is dark blue and clear and filled with light, and each breath you take resonates with the scent of evergreens as the night wind blows through you like angels' voices.

Spring is the time of Passover. A Messianic Rabbi oversees our Seder meal, and I am struck by the prophetic symbolism of the ancient Jewish celebration. As God sent Moses to deliver the Jews from slavery in Egypt, He also sent the Passover Lamb. In Moses' time, the Passover lamb's blood was sprinkled on the doorways of each house, on the top and each side, in the shape of a cross. When the Angel of Death saw the blood, he passed over that house, and all the people in it escaped the great judgment.

Seder tables are covered with white cloths and set with the best silverware, crystal, and china. Candles burn as the Light of God. Bitter herbs, representing suffering, adorn one plate. Sweet apples, representing the joy of deliverance, adorn another. There is special soup and the Passover lamb itself. The unleavened matzah bread is covered by a cloth napkin in a stack of three, and the middle matzah is removed and broken. Red wine in clear glasses is raised at various points in the evening, for a prayer and a toast. Hebrew words and songs entwine the evening. A door is left open, and an empty place is set for the return of the prophet Elijah.

The last toast of the meal is raised with these words:

"Next year in Jerusalem."

How much of all this did Jesus fulfill at His Last Supper—and the days that followed?

One of the best symbols of our mountain unity is the Easter Sunrise service we have every year by the lake. Twelve different churches work together to produce this event, and three hundred people wake up at 5:00 a.m. to be there by 6:00. This year Kristen came up from San Diego to spend the weekend with us and get up early, too. (Ryan didn't make it, but at least he called the night before.)

Edd and his best friend Steve Smith did the music with their talented band. They spent days getting ready, practicing, and setting up sound equipment on the lakeshore. Some of the musicians even camped out the night before to guard their stuff. The other band members got there early and somehow managed to play cold instruments with cold fingers.

And they sang, as the brilliant yellow sunlight topped the tall evergreens and shone on the wind-brushed lake,

"Jesus is Alive!"

And the mountain residents shivered in their blankets and echoed the chorus:

"Jesus is Alive!"

And a lone kayaker paused in his early morning paddle to listen. And a photographer from the valley newspaper took sunrise shots, and the drama team played the women who went to the empty tomb. And a pastor read from the Gospel of John:

> "I am the resurrection and the life;
> he who believes in me,
> though he may die,
> he shall live."

After Jesus was crucified for our sins and buried in a borrowed tomb, can you imagine what that first Easter morning was like? Mary Magdalene, a woman, was the first to go to the tomb and find the guards gone and the huge stone rolled away. She ran to tell Peter and John, the disciples who had been hiding in fear. They came and saw inside the tomb, that the linen cloths that had bound Jesus' body were neatly folded, but Jesus was not there. Can you imagine their amazement as the two men slowly walked back home and discussed the situation? Outside the tomb, Mary waited. She peered in and saw two angels, one at the head, and one at the foot of the empty spot where Jesus' body had been laid. What light shown from inside that tomb—greater than a sunrise!

Mary knelt and cried bitterly, and then Jesus appeared to her and asked, "Woman, why are you weeping?" And she finally recognized Jesus and exclaimed, "Teacher!"

And later Jesus appeared to all the disciples who were hiding behind doors, and He said, "Peace to you! As the Father has sent Me, I also send you." And He breathed on them and said, "Receive the Holy Spirit."

So Jesus gave us the task and power of spreading the Easter resurrection news of hope to a world that so desperately needs it.

After the message, we prayed and listened to people share their testimonies of Christ's power in their lives. Then we gathered up our sandy blankets as the morning sun filled the mountain lake. And we got back into our cars and drove to Lee Johnson's house for his annual pancake and sausage breakfast.

And we sat around his large round table—members of The Band and their families and friends—and we held warm coffee in our warming-up hands and smiled at each other and sang silently, under our breath,

"Jesus is Alive!"

As much as I love these mountains, I realize that they are not separate from the rest of the world. They are tied to the valleys—to the freeways and the pollution and the masses of houses and people stretching from the desert to the sea, from farmland to cities filled with skyscrapers and airports. We who live at six thousand feet drive down the windy roads to work or shop or visit friends. If the cities were destroyed, the mountains would follow. We know this, as Selah did when she stood on the Summit and knew she must return to the valleys.

Today daffodils line the lawns of houses and the edges of forests —huge patches of yellow flowers against dark green. Today the pink, red, and orange tulips crowd into planters, shining with color like sunlight separated into its spectrum. Today the silver fir trees hang down with boughs like lace, new green growth on their fingertip ends.

Today Edd kissed me before leaving early for work (I was still half asleep). His beard rubbed against my cheek, and I wanted to wake up and spend time with him.

Today Jonathan cuddled with me on the sofa, and Jessica drew a picture for me. Today Kristen sent me a greeting card, and Ryan called me on the phone.

Today I am happy to be alive, knowing full well that each day is a gift. If I had lived 200 years ago (or even 50), the cancer would have killed me. (If I had lived 200 years ago, in a less polluted and radioactive world, I probably wouldn't have gotten cancer.)

But my life is full of contrasts, so I realize that—even though I am surrounded by all this spring mountain beauty—I am reminded of loss.

"April is the cruelest month," wrote poet T.S. Elliot, an American who went to live in England. He knew something about not fitting in. He also wrote a poem called "Prufrock," about a shy man who didn't quite fit into society. Prufrock sat on the outside, looking in at life. He "measured out his life with coffee spoons" and dreamed of mermaids swimming in the sea, singing "each to each."

I was born in April, during the Easter season. It is April now, and I think about my life—how I am from the latter part of the 20th century and now part of the 21st. I feel like I was called to be a voice for this generation, this strange world of technology and pollution, of new breakthroughs in medicine and new diseases. Does it matter exactly what year I was born? Isn't the soul timeless, speaking to other souls of other generations, throughout all the Ages?

My minor in college was history, and I feel like a historian, carefully chronicling this Time.

The Apostle Paul warned us not to think of ourselves more highly than we ought to think and to associate with the humble. "Do not be wise in your own opinion," he added (see Romans Chapter 12).

This idea leads me to contemplate the revolutionary heart of the Gospel—that God, even though He made the universe, humbled Himself enough to become a man. He left the Throne of Heaven for a stable, a dusty road, a cross. He lived among us, healed us, let us spit in his face and pound nails into His hands. He bore our sin—that horrible thing that causes suffering and death in our world—and then rose again to give us new life.

And so I have an internal relationship with the Creator, not an external religion of things I must do.

Jesus came not to be served, but to serve. He told us that if we serve The Least of These, we serve Him. A servant's heart is rare.

As Paul said,

"Let each of you look out not only
for his own interests,
but also for the interests of others.

Let this mind be in you
which was also in Christ Jesus,

Who, being in the form of God,
did not consider it robbery
to be equal with God.

But made Himself of no reputation,
taking the form of a bondservant,
and coming in the likeness of men.

And being found in appearance
as a man,
He humbled Himself
and became obedient to the point of death,
even the death of the cross." Philippians 2:5-8

If we really believe this, how will we live? Won't we shout to the world, as Paul did:

> Yet indeed I also count
> all things loss
> for the excellence
> of the knowledge
> of Christ Jesus my Lord,
> for whom I have suffered
> the loss of all things,
> and count them as rubbish,
> that I may gain Christ
>
> And be found in Him,
> not having my own righteousness,
> which is from the law,
> but that which is
> through faith in Christ,
> the righteousness
> which is from God by faith;
>
> That I may know Him
> and the power of His resurrection,
> and the fellowship of His sufferings,
> being conformed to His death,
>
> If, by any means,
> I may attain to the resurrection
> from the dead." Philippians 3:8-11

Paul, like me, lived The Great Adventure. Christianity is not boring, as some people imagine. We don't just sit on hard pews, fall asleep during long sermons, sing old-fashioned songs, and avoid parties. The Bible is not just amazing stories (that don't always show people at their best), poetry, and inspirational thoughts. It's a love letter from our Creator.

My books may not become wildly popular <u>because</u> I am

a Christian. But, hey, would you take Billy Graham or Mother Teresa without Jesus? And think of J.R.R. Tolkien and C.S. Lewis, Christian fantasy writers of the Twentieth Century, who met with other Inklings at an Oxford pub. If I had been one of their group, I would have been the only woman…

So I, like Paul, write for The Least of These—those people like Prufrock who know that April can be the cruelest month, who feel loss instead of gain, death instead of birth, and dreams unfulfilled.

My friend Cherie invited Jess & Jon to her son's sixth birthday party. Since she is pregnant, I wanted to drop the kids off and go do errands so that I didn't have to be around her. But when I walked in the pizza parlor, she invited me to have lunch with them. Since I never could resist free food, I sat down at the long table with the rest of the moms, ate salad, and listened to conversation. Soon the topic turned to Cherie's pregnancy and the trouble she's had so far, including a recent trip to the Emergency Room because of contractions and some bleeding.

"But they checked me and the baby out, and everything seems to be fine," she assured her audience (and herself). "Did I tell you I'm going to have a boy? That means God didn't say 'no' to a boy."

I knew she was referring to the stillborn boy she had two years ago.

Then she turned to look at me and stated,

"Isn't God good?"

My first thought was,

To you, maybe.

And then I thought, God is good whether or not you have this baby boy. Didn't He send His own son to live among us and suffer and die and rise again? Whatever anyone may say about sorrow, God provided the solution in the end.

Then I felt like reminding Cherie that she already had a boy whose birthday we were celebrating, and that she had three girls between the ages of ten and four. I wanted to add that she could still have a miscarriage. I even thought of saying something crass like "don't count your chicks before they hatch." Instead

I realized, sitting there at the pizza parlor with a mouth full of garlic bread, that I had just learned my Biggest Lesson:

It's Not About Me.

Whether I had another baby or not doesn't really matter. My own little desires do not run the universe. There's a whole world of people out there who aren't even surviving, and my focus should go out to them and not inward to myself.

It's like comparing an elite ice rink to a barrio in Tijuana.

My local training rink is on top of a mountain, hidden by a forest, reached only by a narrow, winding road. It is clean and cool and expensive, ice stretched out smooth and ready to be marked by glittering silver blades. The spectators are well dressed and drive nice cars. The skaters wear custom outfits — midnight blue velvet material sewn with crystals, over tights and thousand-dollar skates.

I have worked with various organizations that help poor children, like Spectrum Ministries of San Diego that works in Mexico or Compassion International that supports children all over the world. A Tijuana barrio is miserably hot and dirty. There is no electricity or water, let alone ice. Spectrum has to bring water, tubs, and portable showers to bathe the dirty children who stand by gutted-out buildings. Dogs, covered with scabbies, compete with the humans for food. A child with lice and a skin rash, wearing only colorless, torn shorts and no shoes, stares up at you. Maybe she is missing a limb or has a clef palate. She will never see the inside of an ice rink.

Twenty-Four

Pianos and Parrots

I gave up teaching college English to homeschool our children. Edd has always supported me in this, not pushing me to earn money (good thing, since I can't seem to do that). We turned one bedroom into the School Room, packed full of Impressionist artwork, nature photographs, rock collections, science kits, books, computers and software, videos, art supplies...

I never quite know when we're not homeschooling. Breakfast becomes a cooking lesson. Old Jello becomes an experiment in growing mold as I show the kids white patches suspended throughout the opaque red 3D sphere. The stuff on top is green and fuzzy, and I explain that Penicillin comes from mold.

We examine the structure of a bird's feather, the scales on a butterfly wing, the shape of a snowflake. We make each outing a field trip.

A typical day might be this:

—listen to Edd get up at 5:30 and then drift back to sleep

—pick up my pocket Bible at 8:15 and read a Psalm

—swing my feet over the bed to touch the floor by 8:30, and my nonstop day begins

—tape <u>Battlestar Galactica</u> from the Sci Fi channel only to discover that the first episode and a half didn't work because I set the VCR wrong

—do Math with Jessica at the kitchen table and Writing

with Jonathan at his desk in the computer room, running back and forth as each child needs help

—call 10 different people or agencies on the phone (thank God for headsets)
—check emails
—do History with Jessica and Reading with Jonathan
—collect poop samples for the lab (Jessie's having stomach problems)
—take a quick shower
—give Jess a Spelling test while Jonathan does Math in his workbook
—drop Jonathan at Blake's house
—drive down the mountain to the medical building
—check in at the allergist for Jessica
—take poop samples to the lab in the basement
—rush to the other side of the building and check in with my doctor (I'm double-booked again)
—go back to the allergist and stay with Jessica while she gets all those scratches on her back
—return to my doctor when we're done at the allergist
—leave the medical building and drive to Costco for shopping and gas
—find <u>Battlestar Galactica</u> on DVD at Costco
—drive back up the mountain
—pick up Jonathan
—rush home to make dinner, Edd's morning coffee, and his lunch
—eat, clean the table, and do dishes while Edd grades papers and Jess and Jon show him their homeschool work
—wonder how I'm going to finish my books, find a better publisher, and get a literary agent
—read a Psalm to the kids before tucking them into bed

Jonathan is like a sponge, taking in everything. Yet in many ways, he is still my baby. At seven, he follows me around the house and cuddles with me (even to the point of annoying when he sits in my lap and grabs me around my neck). I hold him, and his eyes grow sleepy as I stroke his curly hair and wrap my fingers around his slender wrists.

Jonathan is my "Gift from God," as his Hebrew name means. He is a friend, like Prince Jonathan, son of King Saul, was a friend to the shepherd boy named David. David was the youngest of his brothers, stuck out in the fields and forgotten. Yet <u>he</u> was the one called by Samuel the Prophet and anointed to be the future King. David probably had curly, reddish hair and beautiful eyes, and he wrote poetry and songs that later became half the book of Psalms. David played stringed instruments, and when mad King Saul heard about it, he called David to his palace to play for him:

"The Lord is my shepherd;
I shall not want..."

until the King's troubled soul was eased. For all his help, Saul became jealous of David when he killed the giant Philistine named Goliath (now that's a story!), and all the women sang praise to David. Even though Saul gave David his own daughter in marriage, the King still hated him. One night, in a fit of rage, King Saul threw his spear at David and nearly pinned him to the wall.

Jonathan, by birthright, would have been the next King of Israel. But he knew that God had chosen David instead. Yet Jonathan was faithful to his friend and protected him from his father's madness. He sent David off to the wilderness to hide from his father. And Jonathan came out secretly to the desert to encourage David.

King Saul hunted David for years, and David had to stay in caves, forests, foreign countries, and lonely mountains. Even when given the chance, David would not strike at Saul. He waited for God's judgment. It came in a battle against the Philistines. When Jonathan was killed in the battle next to his father, David wrote a song to remember his friend:

"How the mighty have fallen

in the midst of the battle!
Jonathan was slain in your high places.

I am distressed for you,
my brother Jonathan;
You have been very pleasant to me;
Your love to me was wonderful..." 2 Samuel 1:25 & 26

My Jonathan was born to me through cancer and pain. When he was newborn he slept on my chest. When he was older he slept in the crib next to my bed and would slip his small hands through the cribslats to hold mine.

He is a beautiful child. Since his curly hair, expressive eyebrows, and blue eyes make him look just like Frodo from <u>The Lord of the Rings</u>, he dreams of traveling to New Zealand. He wants to see where the films were made and meet Elijah Wood. Wherever we go, people say, "Oh, he is so adorable" or "he looks like he could be in that movie..."

"I want to be an actor," he tells me again.

He makes homeschool full of wonder as he sparks passion for learning. He sets up his own laboratory in the back yard, using any old containers and food dye I don't want. He's learning to write down the ingredients of his experiments. He took a science class from another homeschool dad and got so excited over electricity and circuits that "Mr. Science" joked about him being the one to blow up the science lab. I dreamed all night about keeping him away from electrical outlets and powerlines—forces he does not fully understand.

"I want to be a scientist," he informs me.

Ever since he was a few months old, he could hum melodies perfectly in tune. When he was two, we bought him a little portable keyboard, and he carried it with him everywhere and plopped down to pick at the keys, learning songs by ear, like his father does. I'll watch Jonathan stand behind his father who plays on his full-size keyboard. Jonathan is smiling as he listens to Edd finger each key. His little hand rests on Edd's shoulder as morning sunlight pours through the window onto their faces and mingles with the high-pitched notes.

"I want to be a musician like you, and lead worship in church," he tells Edd.

Jonathan and I do our Community Bible Studies together. He sits in my lap and kisses me periodically. I read the New King James words, and his eyes and voice follow along as he traces his finger next to mine upon the text. He slowly writes out sentences under typed questions on his paper. Then he proudly takes his little Bible to the drug store and, while waiting in line with me, reads from 1 Corinthians 13, so that the grandparents standing behind us are impressed and say that God must be calling him for a great work.

"I want to be a preacher," he promises.

Jonathan has always been my comforter, as if he knows what I have suffered.

When he's not cuddling with me, Jonathan writes me little notes on yellow paper (in his shaky beginning handwriting),

I love you,
Jon

If I go away on a women's retreat for the weekend, when I return he sits in my lap and says,

"I missed you. I smelled you in my shirt. I'm so glad you survived cancer. I would have missed you so much."

When I'm cooking, he wanders into the kitchen, smells the pot on the stove, and says,

"That looks like it will make me sick. Especially if it's made by Mama."

I give him chores to do. It was his idea to vacuum, and at first he loved to push around the vacuum cleaner that is almost as tall as he is. Then the chore became work, and he no longer wanted to do it.

"Why do I have to vacuum?" he asks me, frowning, one hand on the vacuum cleaner handle.

"Because it's your job," I reply.

"Then fire me," he retorts.

I laugh, of course, but I make him continue vacuuming.

He gets me back a few days later when he overhears me saying I am going to write about him and his vacuuming job.

"I don't want to be in your dumb book!" he yells, partly mad at me, partly embarrassed that his privacy is being invaded.

I bend down and explain that it is an honor to be written into a book.

His critique humbles me, though he does change his mind later and allows me to put his story in my book.

He still runs everywhere he goes. When he scoots outside, he pauses to turn and look at me. Sunlight filters through cedars above him, their branches spread like green lace. His face is a mix of light and shadow. His eyes are blue fire beneath his random curls. He waves, then runs up stone steps and into the forest. Like a hobbit, he disappears among the trees.

Let me live to see Jonathan grown, with children of his own, I pray.

Jessica is quiet and thoughtful. She finds lost fledglings every spring and picks up the baby birds as if she were born to work with them, holding them on her finger and speaking to them, calming them with her soft voice. She helped my friend Mary Pat raise orphaned baby bluebirds, placing worms into their open beaks. Jessica can work on her own, spending all day researching snow leopards or parrots.

Parrots live in the Amazon rain forest which teems with life in all directions—trees, vines, ferns, flowers, animals, insects. Parrots chatter together in treetops, eat fruit and seeds, drink from white flowers cupped with rain, and stretch their wings against the sky. Parrots see in more colors than we do, easily recognizing each other's feather patterns in iridescent shades of green, yellow, blue, orange, pink, red.

Parrots mate for life. They stay together constantly, preening each other, bonding so strongly that if one dies, the other may follow. Parrots bond to their human the same way, so if they are left for even a few days, they can die. Parrots love to play and be petted, curiously examining any new object offered to them.

Jessica is like a parrot, always needing her social calendar filled with activities and friends. "I want to be a bird trainer when I grow up," she kept telling us, so we bought her a Senegal parrot for her tenth birthday. Its ancestors come from the jungles of West Africa. It is plump and bigger than a blue jay, its feathers shades of living green, from neon to olive, with yellow and peach underneath and gray on top of her head. Penny loves Jessica and is content to sit on her shoulder and rub against her cheek.

Jessie has seen an African Gray, the most intelligent of all parrots, at the Wild Animal Park. "Bruce Nadell" could talk really well, answering the random commands of his trainer. African Grays speak with understanding. They are sensitive and creative and need so much attention that if neglected or abused, they can pluck out their own feathers. Isn't this like some humans who show self-destructive behavior because of the pain in their life? Isn't this like rejected writers?

Jess visited an African Gray last night, at a neighbor's house. "Baby" lives in the garage, and the owner would like to sell her to a home where she could have more attention. Jess held the large parrot, about two years old, who perched perfectly still on her hand and studied her with bright blue eyes against beautiful silver feathers edged with white, a scalloped pattern more intricate than any artist could reproduce. I imagined an African Gray in my Junior Bird Trainer's future, as she stood there with her hair trailing down her back like Arwen the elf princess. I imagine that the elves in The Lord of the Rings can speak to birds.

But Jessie will probably have to wait for her African Gray, since Baby costs $800 dollars and we also have little Penny the Senegal parrot. Maybe if I could sell more books...

Jessie is strong and muscular, tall for her age. She takes skating seriously, urging me to be on time for lessons, warming up to Yoga videos, and practicing her jumps and spins in the living room. She likes to read her American Girl magazine, curled up on the sofa, her Kirsten doll (with freshly braided blonde hair), sitting next to her. She understands how I sometimes crave time to myself, like she does (hard to do with an annoying little brother).

I buy her art books, and when she is not sketching birds, she draws cartoons of girls in frustrating situations, capturing the slanted frown and bright eyes of a ten-year-old. Her sense of humor and sarcasm are keen, and she told me once (after watching the orthopedic surgeon cut off my cast to show the 13 staples under it):

"I know one thing. When I grow up, I want nothing to do with the medical profession."

She remembers little of me going through cancer, but that experience probably helped her decide against being a doctor.

Jessica writes letters, getting one published in American Girl magazine. Maybe she'll be a writer like me...

She loves to read, surrounding herself with books and magazines. She enjoys my books because:

"they create a world inside my head."

As she speaks, her long auburn hair hangs past her bottom, curling in ringlets on the ends. She is wearing her usual skating outfit of black leggings and a red top. Her eyes look bigger behind her pink metallic eyeglasses. Holding a book in one hand, she adds:

"You can learn a lot from reading."

Twenty-Five

To the Future

Today at church I sit beside Doris, our mountain naturalist. She could have been my mother if she'd had me by the time she was twenty.

She is still fighting her melanoma.

Life is full of setbacks. You start feeling better, and then you feel worse again. Able to identify with that feeling, I ask her how she is doing. She tells me, tears close behind her light blue eyes. She bows her white head with me as I lay my hand on her shoulder and pray for her.

You have to be wounded yourself—and then healed—to be a healer.

I wander out to the church steps and watch the children play with left-over balloons (Edd, who has been leading worship music, is putting equipment away). The children tie their balloons all together with white ribbons and come up with a plan of letting them loose. With giggles and yells, they stand in a line with their balloons and then release them. Immediately the mountain wind picks them up and carries them above the slope, above the tallest pine trees. Red, yellow, white, and pink circles shrink smaller and smaller in the sky. I imagined that they will soar over the mountain top, across the desert on the other side, and up to heaven.

I feel sad at the sight, as if the balloons are the souls of children who will grow up and fly away.

Jonathan, shorter than the other kids and wearing his red

sweater that makes his blonde curls glow, changes his mind about the whole project. Whining because his balloons are gone, he runs toward the slope as if he can get them back.

Let them go, I think. They are free, riding on the wind.

Like we release balloons into the air, we release our children. A year after my chemo treatments, Kristen visited us before going back to high school in Washington:

"To the Future"

Early in the morning after Edd has gone to work, Kristen opens the computer room door and heads for the bathroom. She's wearing her pink "coffee bean" pajamas which match my long nightgown. I put the kettle on the stove and hear a knock on the door. It's Beth, Kristen's best friend. She has come to say goodbye to Kristen who must return to Washington.

"Hi, Beef," Kristen says, calling Beth by her nickname.

"Hi, Nick," Beth replies. She hands Kristen a going-away card, and they sit cross-legged together on the computer room floor among Kristen's sleeping bag and suitcase that spills over with clothes and books.

(This time she brought some Classics and her Student Bible. "Mom, I'll never get any sleep in here, surrounded by all these great books," she told me when she first set down her suitcase. "Could you spare a copy of Dante's Inferno?")

I spy on the two eighteen-year-olds, both about to launch into their college lives, careers, eventual marriages, and motherhood (or so they hope). They look at old photographs together, giggling.

Seeing me, Beth holds up the famous "Black and White Photo" I took when the two girls first met—at church shortly after Kristen came to live with us when they were both fifteen. Kristen, rebellious, wore a short, velvet black dress with black nylons and black high-heeled shoes. In the photo, she stood stiffly, her hair crimped, too much mascara on her eyelashes, and large gold hoops in her ears. Beth, dressed in a calf-length white dress with a lacy collar, no makeup or jewelry, and white stockings with flat shoes, leaned slightly toward Kristen, her hand held outward as she spoke.

"This is a great picture, isn't it?" Beth asks.

They show me their prom photos, both wearing the same pink ballroom gown with its full taffeta skirt and long sash. They both curled their hair and pinned it atop their heads. They both looked like princesses for one night.

Now, two blonde heads bend toward each other. Make-up free, in pastel cotton clothes, they seem like sisters exchanging secret gifts. They wipe away stray tears and clasp their hands to say goodbye.

"You'll be back for Christmas, won't you?" Beth asks as she searches her purse for a tissue.

"I hope so," Kristen replies, handing Beth a Kleenex.

They both smile and giggle again, each a little afraid of the future—like I am as I stand in the hallway and spy.

Oh Lord, I pray as I return to the whistling teapot on the stove. I'm married to a good man. My two little ones have a long way to go until they're grown. Kristen won't always live in Washington...

Why am I so afraid? I'm afraid of growing too old and outliving everyone, of dying young and leaving my family, of getting pregnant again, of not getting pregnant again, of more separations and illness and change and grief...Help me to trust that You are Lord of the Future as well as the Present and Past. I see how You've walked with me this far, how my life has unfolded like a pattern that makes sense. Surely You can do the same with the unborn years...

I stare at the teakettle for a moment, bright stainless steel fogged by the steam forced from its mouth. The sound hits a high note, a kind of sorrowful wail.

O God, I don't want Jessica and Jonathan to grow up too. I don't want to bury Edd as Ginny and Beverly buried their husbands this year. I don't want to grow a tumor inside me again...Help me to stop feeling like something bad will happen, some tragedy or phone call waiting on the other side of a door...

I stare at my refrigerator which has so many colorful magnets and photos on it that you can't tell it's white. In the center, on a green piece of paper, reads a quote my cousin Stanley from North Carolina sent me:

"Don't be afraid of tomorrow;
God is already there."

A verse from Revelation Chapter 21 seeps into my mind, words that Christ spoke concerning the New Heaven and New Earth:

"Behold, I make all things new...
I am the Alpha and the Omega,
the Beginning and the End.
I will give of the fountain of the water of life
freely to him who thirsts."

I pour the steaming water into three ceramic cups. I will fill one cup with apple herb tea for Beth, one with strong coffee for Kristen, and one with English Breakfast tea for me. While Jessica and Jonathan still sleep, we three women will sit at the dining table to share a prayer and a toast—
to the future.

Twenty-Six

" *** Christians"

I go to my first big book convention, The Christian Book Association Annual Bookfair in Anaheim. <u>Selah of the Summit</u> just got published, and I need to promote it (and maybe find a bigger publisher). It's a two-hour drive one way to Anaheim. Edd takes a day off to stay home with the children. My publisher, GreatUnpublished (aka Booksurge), has sent Stephanie all the way from Charleston to meet me there and promote books by some of GU's inspirational authors.

I had to make a lot of phone calls to get a pass to this bookfair, since the publisher sharing its booth with us was reluctant to issue me a badge. I know I've been a pest, but I am a cancer survivor and don't take "no" easily. This is a big universe. There is always a way. "Never give up; never surrender."

As I drive down, Stephanie calls me on my cellphone to say she has my badge and is standing out front so that I won't have to wait in line for an hour to get it.

"Thanks!" I say as I pull off the freeway. I follow the map I downloaded from the CBA website, pay my $8.00 for parking, find a spot near some stairs, and walk toward the huge, flag-dotted Anaheim Convention Center.

After a couple of cell-to-cell calls, Stephanie and I find each other among the crowd. She is wearing a green dress with a shell necklace. She looks just like the picture she emailed me: shoulder-length red hair, green eyes, a few freckles.

"Hey, Lonna!" she says as we embrace.

I've been emailing Stephanie and talking to her on the phone for two years, so I feel like I know her.

"I know I've been aggressive about getting here," I admit as we walk toward the entrance, badges on. "Sometimes it's a fine line between being ambitious and obnoxious. But I've found that I've got to be aggressive to get anything done. I basically do it out of desperation. Sometimes that puts people off—especially men."

"That's OK," Stephanie replies, showing her badge to the attendant. "People often think I'm younger than I am, and they don't take me as seriously as they should."

I nod as we walk briskly toward Booth 914 where we are sharing a spot with another publisher.

We find a large booth with three tables, bookshelves, chair, a big display, and several people standing around in black suits. I'm not kidding. Black. Scenes from the film <u>Men in Black</u> run through my mind.

"I'm sorry, but we have no room for you," the president of the publishing company tells us.

"But I thought we were sharing this booth," Stephanie replies.

"I'm sorry, but we have no room."

I look at the space in the booth and decide that it could easily hold another table. They've put a large table in the middle where their many authors will sit, smiling, getting their photo taken under a "Meet the Author" banner.

"No problem," I whisper to Stephanie as we walk away, perplexed. "I'll go to the convention people and get another table. I know it's possible to put a small one in that corner."

We approach the president with this idea and he says,

"No, we will not authorize another table. Here, we will give you this corner of a shelf."

His assistant has cleared away a tiny spot that will maybe hold five titles. I glance back at the center table, the large rectangular one for their authors, and realize there is no spot for me.

Stephanie and I walk away again.

"Just let me handle the booth, Lonna," she says in her "calm down and don't be pushy" tone. "I don't want to offend them. We're obviously not even welcome to stand here. You can take some of your books and walk the floor. I'll set out some books and then do the same."

"If they won't let us have our own table, that's OK," I say. "I'm sorry about their attitude, Stephanie."

" *** Christians," Stephanie says under her breath.

"Hey, we're not all like that," I reply. "I think this company is using the term 'Christian' lightly. In fact, I think there's much here at this convention that is not Christian. Obviously the idea of sharing has missed its mark. If Jesus were to walk in, which he couldn't do without a badge or a miracle, the attendants would probably try to throw Him out because He didn't meet the dress code."

She nods, and I reach out and touch her arm. I want to show her that Christians, of all people, should be kind and creative, attractive and witty, joyful and giving. Will she see Jesus in me? How true is the saying "You are the only Jesus some people will ever see"?

Stephanie may never read <u>Crossing the Chemo Room</u> or this sequel. She may only read my actions as I briefly interact with her life.

"I don't mind wandering around the floor like a homeless person," I say with a smile. "I'll get us some free samples!"

"I'll go get the box of books," Stephanie decides, shaking a little with controlled anger. "But first I'm going to find a Starbucks. I need a cup of coffee to calm my nerves."

We separate. I don't know where to start or exactly what to do, so I go to the far left end of the huge convention floor and start walking by publisher booths. I've got my heavy briefcase slung over my right shoulder and a stack of books, information sheets, business cards, and order forms cradled in my left arm. One booth gives me a free book bag, and I start collecting company keychains, flashlights, business cards, sample books, and water bottles.

After a few minutes of this, I pause in one large center booth. A friendly attendant comes to chat with me.

"I just want to rest," I whine. "I thought I had some space in a booth, but I don't."

"You can sit here," he offers. He pushes a chair toward me and gives me a free book. I show him my three.

"Maybe you could order some for your chain of bookstores," I suggest, handing him the appropriate forms.

"Thanks; I'll look these over. So you didn't have any space to set them out?"

"Just part of a little corner shelf, down low."

"Well, that's better than nothing. God can use a little corner shelf. People will come by and take free samples."

"Yeah, I guess, but I feel like a wanderer here with not so much as a chair of my own."

"Jesus had no place to lay His head. And remember that there wasn't even room for Him in the Inn when He was about to be born into this crowded world."

I stare at the booth attendant for a moment. He's a black man in a white-collared shirt with his company's name sewn on it.

"Yeah, I guess you're right. God can use a little corner shelf and a wanderer like me."

I get up, gather my pile of stuff to carry, and head on toward the even bigger booths. One of them, Tyndale House, is where I wouldn't mind my books being published. They have a huge booth with cushioned chairs and a bar offering coffee and chocolate. I've sent query letters to them twice, and twice I've received a form letter telling me how to send a query letter.

Basically, I need a good literary agent or a referral from one of their authors. It's who you know that counts in any business world, and the "Christian" one is harder to break into than the secular one. I decide to hang out in the Tyndale booth and hope to meet one of their famous authors whose names and photos decorate their expensive temporary walls. This booth must have cost them $60,000 for three days...

I actually do meet a couple of authors who even take a

copy of my books. Maybe they'll remember me...I'm wearing my black dress with tan sugar cane reeds on it, that I bought in Kauai last year. I've also got on the big white Mother of Pearl necklace with matching earrings that Edd bought for me in the open-air market. With lots of cross necklaces here, I figure a big pearly shell will be more remembered...

From my spot I can see next door to a music company's booth. It has a big, clear plastic tube out front with a wind tunnel in it and dollar bills floating around. "Catch the Cash" reads the sign above it, and a person stands there to urge someone to get in the tube and catch some cash.

"I don't need money that badly," someone behind me murmurs. I think that, if Jesus walked by here, He would chase these cash people out with a whip as He did when He found the moneychangers in the Temple.

"This is my Father's House, a House of Prayer, but you have made it a den of thieves," He told them.

There is much here that is not Christian. Business is business, driven by profit. And yet here I am, trying to find a bigger publisher, trying to get orders for my books. Do I want my name and photo plastered on a wall? Do I want to sit at a draped table while people wait in line to get my autograph?

When I had a book signing at my local library, though it was announced in the local papers, very few people came. If I were J.K. Rowling, there would have been masses...

One man sat in front. He wore ragged jeans and torn tennis shoes. His shirt was not new. His hair was long and straggly, brown with streaks of gray. He asked me about writing and then bought one of my books with ten crinkly dollars that were stuffed in his pocket—all that he had.

He was not handsome or cocky like the man in the back who enjoyed debating with Christians. But I felt honored that he had come to my book signing. James, the practical disciple who told us to be doers of the word and not hearers only, warned us against showing partiality to the well-dressed, wealthy person and ignoring the poor man...

An announcement on the loudspeaker brings me back to

the CBA Bookfair. A couple of the well-dressed writers wander toward me. They have tailored beige suits, designer glasses, and polished leather shoes. The man's hair is newly styled above his monogrammed collar, and the woman has heavy make-up, puffy bleached hair, and high heels. I stare at them and wonder what it means to be a writer. Is it the big name that everyone recognizes above the professionally-shot black and white photo? Is it the million-dollar advance from a large publishing house, the number of people lined up to meet you, the bodyguards, the fake smile? Or is it simply the act of writing, what we do in secret, alone at a keyboard, typing each word out, one painful letter at a time?

As I sit and watch the Tyndale House writers mingle in their expensive booth, helping themselves to Godiva chocolates and Starbucks coffee, I realize that you've got to balance <u>living</u> with writing. Don't just shut yourself in a room with a keyboard. Live your life. Write what you know first; then you can create amazing new worlds in far-away galaxies. Don't forget what is most important—the people you love. Their souls will far outlast your words. If you're married, don't neglect your husband's dinner, morning coffee, or need to talk at 2:00 a.m. If you're a mother, write while your children play at your feet (and don't get too angry if they unplug the computer before you saved your words). Or write on your laptop while you half watch a soccer game or on notepads while waiting at the doctor's office. Put your family into your writing. Let them sit at a booth and help you sell books. Make them part of your writing life.

I think, more than anything, that a writer writes out of personal pain—to understand suffering and transform it to beauty.

Artists do the same. My friend Mary Smith has a fourteen-year-old daughter named Chelsea. Chelsea has Crohn's disease and spent the summer in the Pediatric Intensive Care Unit of a hospital, hooked up to I.V.s because she could not eat or drink. The doctors didn't know what to do and thought they might lose her. Mary stayed with her daughter constantly, camping out every night in that small hospital room, on a hideaway bed, making sure the nurses did their best when drawing Chelsea's blood, weighing her, or checking for internal bleeding.

My new church (we're going to Calvary Chapel now) sent the elders to pray for Chelsea and anoint her with oil. She started improving. The doctors began giving her liquids and unhooking her I.V.s. Chelsea started using her time in the hospital. She hand-painted wooden boxes and plaques and soon had enough inventory to cover a hospital table. Doctors and nurses stopped by to purchase the handmade gifts.

Chelsea made something lovely out of her pain. She even practiced calligraphy, covering her walls with scripture verses bordered by pastel flowers.

For me, writing is worship—time alone with God, reading the Bible, weaving God's words into the story He has made of my life...

One of the Tyndale staff has noticed me sitting in the overstuffed chair for too long. She walks up and asks, in that "who are you and what are you doing here" tone:

"May I help you?"

I get the hint, gather up my armful of stuff, and move on.

There is much at this bookfair that is showy and secular, I think as I watch the bustle around me. Yet there is something here that is Christian. I have a heavy bag full of things people have given me. I've been invited to sit in people's booths, and, when I was having an anxiety attack after all the stress and walking and presenting my books with a sales pitch, one man named Gabriel brought me a cold water bottle. He was kind and softspoken and took my book descriptions, promising to send them on to his publisher's acquisitions editor. He asked me if I was all right and checked on me during the ten minutes I sat on his company's sofa, my face red and my heart pounding.

If I ever do see my books widely distributed, I hope it is not just to Christian bookstores. If people come to recognize my name, I hope it points to Jesus.

Toward the end of the day, I find a "Lord of the Rings" display by Houghton Mifflin, a publisher I have been sending query letters to for years. They are not just Christian, but publish a wide variety of books. The rep and I start conversing about the differences between Harry Potter and Frodo, and she seems impressed by my observations. She takes a copy of <u>Selah of the Summit</u> and asks me to email her in a week.

As I walk away, I think maybe a door is starting to open. Jesus told his disciples:

"Ask, and it will be give to you;
Seek, and you will find;
knock, and it will be opened to you." (Matthew 7:7)

He didn't say exactly when this would happen, or where.
Like Selah, I stand before a door as it moves on its hinges. I have been beating on this door until I've just about broken it down. Just ask Stephanie about that. And even if a big, important door doesn't open for me through this CBA Bookfair, at least I've met Stephanie and have shared the experience with her. For months afterward we can send each other emails, joking about "Mr. Jerk" who wouldn't share his booth with us—and about what names Jesus used for religious hypocrites. And I'll send a report to GreatUnpublished co-founder Jeff Schwaner, who first gave my words shape, and thank him for the publishing revolution that can fly against the long-established companies and give the rest of us a chance.

And if the door opens, should I go through? What waits on the other side? Maybe I'm finally learning that they're God's books, not mine. The words are a gift. They can make even me cry. If they weren't so Christian, maybe they'd win an award...

In The Book of Revelation, Jesus said to the church at Philadelphia:

"These things says He who is holy,
He who has the key of David,
He who opens and no one shuts,
and shuts and no one opens"
I know your works.
See, I have set before you

an open door..." (Revelation 3:7)

In <u>The Lord of the Rings</u>, Frodo went through doors. Some were pleasant, as in the House of Elrond at Rivendell where white-carved Elven halls sheltered him among waterfalls and trees in the mountains. Some doors were horrible like the tall iron door in the Mines of Moria. Beneath it lay a stone tomb, the bodies of dwarves, and a fiery demon.

May I have the wisdom to know which door to knock on, which door to walk through, which door God is opening.

And, like Frodo, may I always remember that I am ordinary. Though my quest may succeed and though my name may become known, I will always bear the scars of the long, long journey.

Twenty-Seven

Crying in MiMi's Cafe

This year has been a struggle health-wise. I've had more pain, sleeplessness, and specialist appointments than since I had cancer. My allergies act up and my sinuses go berserk, especially when there's a wildfire nearby, which is common in dry California. I get The Virus of the Week from my mountain friends or family. But my doctors tell me my health is pretty good:

"Wings of an Eagle"

I found a new oncologist and got my overdue checkup, enduring exams, bloodwork, x-rays, mammograms, and a CAT-scan.

Before getting my CAT-scan, feeling nervous and scared, I wanted a Valium. But since I had no one to drive me back up the mountain, the hospital told me they wouldn't give me one. Instead, I drove by the church on my way "down the hill." A couple of elders happened to be there on that Friday afternoon, and they prayed for me and anointed me with oil.

This was better than Valium. I felt greatly honored, for the New Testament sick were anointed with oil, and the kings of Israel were anointed with oil:

"You anoint my head with oil;
my cup runs over." (Psalm 23:5)

I had to wait an hour and 15 minutes to get into the CAT-scan room, so I spent the time chatting with patients and giving a copy of <u>Crossing the Chemo Room</u> to an Oncology nurse. When my turn finally came, I didn't mind the dye the technician put in my veins via an I.V. or the awful white liquid he gave me to drink. The tube and laser lights and holding my breath brought back memories from six years ago, but it was over in 15 minutes.

Two weeks later, I went in to the oncologist to get my test results. I had to take deep breaths as the doctor repeated my long medical history. When he finally told me my recent test results, they were all, amazingly, normal.

Then something weird happened. Dr. Rentchler showed me the CAT-scan report of six years ago. There, in black letters under the date and my name, were some sentences about abnormal lumps in both my kidneys.

"From where I'm standing, it looks like the lymphoma had spread to your kidneys, and you were in Stage IV of the disease, not Stage I," he told me.

He was short and bald (appropriate for working with chemotherapy), with startling blue eyes like an eagle's. Nothing like the tall, dark-haired, brown-eyed Dr. Schinke.

"But Dr. Schinke told me the CAT-scan was clear, and that I was in Stage I," I replied, amazed. "How can this be?"

"It's a mystery. Your recent CAT-scan was normal—nothing odd in your kidneys or anywhere else. The chemo must have zapped the lymphoma in your kidneys. Or perhaps there was some mistake in the original test. In any case, you are cured."

I stared at the eagle pictures and statues lining Dr. Rentchler's exam room. In the window, a stained glass eagle spread its wings above one of my favorite Bible verses:

"Those who wait on the LORD
Shall renew their strength;
They shall mount up with wings like eagles,
They shall run and not be weary,
They shall walk and not faint." (Isaiah 40:31)

"I like that verse," I told the matter-of-fact oncologist. He smiled and held out his hand to shake mine.

"Thank you," I said in a low voice. Then I turned past the double doors of another Chemo Room that I would not have to enter.

As I drove up the mountain from the doctor's office, still stunned from a medical report of six years ago, I realized that, if that report were correct, that makes me even more of a miracle...

I will sometimes want to hide away on my mountain and never see a doctor again. But I will realize that I cannot cut myself off from the medical community. They are part of me now. They brought me through cancer and will now help me deal with the long-term effects of the cure.

Besides, I must eat my own words.

I wrote that battling cancer is like fighting The Alien. Those words were published in my local county newspaper, and people have read them. Those words are in this book. I cannot deny them.

When you go hiking in the forest at twilight and come across a mountain lion, what do you do?

The worst thing is to turn and run. The cougar will chase after you and attack you from behind with his powerful claws and teeth. The second worst thing is to ignore the lion. He will sense your fear and stalk you. You must stand tall, raise your arms, yell, and look threatening. Then the giant cat will leave you alone.

And cancer is far worse than a mountain lion. It is worse even than The Alien in horror films. You cannot run; you cannot hide. Face the monster. Fight. Those medical tests and doctors are your allies in the battle.

So I will visit doctors' offices and hospitals, talking to cancer patients and giving away my books, feeling a little like Mother Teresa bringing hope to the sick.

But my resolve doesn't always stand firm. Sometimes I feel like bursting into tears.

I did just that in, of all places, MiMi's Cafe:

"Crying in MiMi's Cafe"

A few months after the Christian Booksellers Association Bookfair, I didn't see any doors opening. All the emails and letters and free books that I sent out to my "contacts" from that bookfair had been ignored or rejected, increasing my large collection of "dear author" letters, and I heard from none of the famous authors who might have given me a referral.

One afternoon I went "down the hill" to shop at Costco (of course, bringing both kids with me). Afterward, we went to MiMi's cafe, one of my favorite places.

Let me tell you a few things about MiMi's. Its Mocha Latte (with Ghirardelli chocolate) can cure most forms of depression—at least temporarily. It comes in a big round crockery bowl painted bright yellow. It is topped with whipped cream, and you need a spoon to get the full effect. I figure that Heaven will have something like a MiMi's Cafe.

My best friend Mary Pat, whom I met at a Parents' Night Out dinner dance when we first moved to the mountains, also loves MiMi's. She is like me: creative and eccentric, from a difficult childhood, with no family nearby. She has reddish brown hair, hazel eyes, and glasses. She reminds me of Anne Shirley from the <u>Anne of Green Gables</u> books—abt to speak her mind and get in trouble for it, but always risking an adventure.

Mary Pat and I have been known to take two-hour lunches at MiMi's, surrounded by three children (her daughter Kaley is five), French Onion soup, and glasses of iced tea with lemon. We sit at our red-checked booth, chatting and browsing over mail-order catalogs while the sun lowers toward the west outside a cheerful French-style window. The window has a real wooden sill, painted rustic green, and a rooster statue on the shelf below it. Nearby is the Cappuccino Bar, with mugs and glasses hanging on the wall above it and little brass lamps set along a marble counter. People can unwind there, lounging on tall barstools as friendly servers take their order and show them poppy seed muffins from the bakery display.

But on this particular day Mary Pat wasn't with me, and Edd was working. It was hot outside, with a Santa Anna wind blowing from the eastern deserts and threatening another wildfire (we had one on our mountainside last June, and the thick red cloud of smoke and ash made us, for the first time, consider leaving the mountain). I had a difficult week of doctor's appointments, homeschool, figure skating schedules, Internet endeavors, bill-juggling, trying to work on this book, and dealing with tenants who won't pay rent (lesson learned: never rent anything to anyone). I made the mistake of bringing a book catalog with me to MiMi's—a big, full-color one from a well-known Christian bookstore chain. As I waited for my mocha latte, I started glancing through the pages of well-advertised books.

Before I knew it, tears were rolling down my cheeks. Jessica stared at me, and Jonathan patted my hand.

"Look at this!" I told them, their surprised faces watching me point to the color photos of books, with titles and authors in bold black letters. "All these people get help selling their books. And many of them don't even have much talent! Who cares about a book on Christian home decorating or <u>What Would Jesus Eat</u>? How can something with the word "Hug" in the title be a Best Seller? Why is a teapot sold at a Christian store? When did so much fluffy merchandise take over, while writers like me, who have written for years—with all their heart and their own life's blood—get ignored by the big publishing companies who dare to call themselves Christian—the doors slammed in our faces, like it must have been for Mary and Joseph at the Bethlehem Inn?"

I blew my nose loudly on my mint green cloth napkin.

"It just depends on who you know. It's a big Members Only Club, and I'm tired of trying to beat down the door."

"Well, I like your <u>Selah</u> book," Jessie said in her soft voice, her long auburn braid bobbing a little as she shook her head. "I feel like going to those publishing companies and yelling at them to publish your books."

"Yeah," Jonathan repeated, one eyebrow raised over his

big blue seven-year-old eyes. He was wearing his Stained Glass Window sweater even though it was warm outside.

The hot tears still coursed annoyingly down my face. I picked up my red cell phone, pressed one of the buttons so that the green backlight would come on, and set it back down on the blue tablecloth.

"Many of the great writers never saw their words in print or never made any money by them," I lectured as if to an English class. "Remember how I told you about one of my favorite poets, Emily Dickinson? She never got married or had kids. She saw very few of her words in print though she wrote hundreds of little poems, sewed them neatly into packets, and hid them in her drawers. Now, over a hundred years after her death, her work is known and loved all over the world. There are Emily Dickinson Societies. High school and college classes require students to read her poems.

"But I'm no Emily Dickinson. I'd like to make money to help pay off our bills."

I threw the catalog into a corner and stared at it, then continued my lecture. "Remember how we rearranged our Classic Books in our home library last week, and I picked up an old copy of Paradise Lost by John Milton?"

"Yes," Jessie replied. "I remember seeing your poetry book, too."

I hardly ever think about my old Master's thesis in its green hardbound cover with gold letters on the spine and a total printing of 3 copies. I pretty much gave up writing poetry to craft poetic nonfiction.

"I remember how I sat cross-legged next to you on the floor," Jessica continued.

I must have surprised her that afternoon when I suddenly started crying as I held the Milton book like an old, neglected friend and slowly ran my finger over the red leather cover, ridged spine, and gilt-edged pages. I opened the book and looked at reproductions of the black-and-white woodcuts by the famous romantic poet William Blake. I read aloud the first page of the tragic saga of The Fall of Man, then held up Blake's tormented picture of an angel driving out Adam and Eve. The beautiful Seventeenth Century English poetic verse and Eighteenth Century images filled the dusty room of books, computers, and artwork where we did our homeschool.

"I used to have time to read books," I wept then as I closed Milton.

"I will read that book someday," Jessica promised me.

And I knew that the Internet and electronic formats and handheld computers will never replace a good old dusty book with real paper pages. And though my own books have forms as cute paperbacks or Internet downloads, they are not in this glossy catalog or the shelves of bookstores across the world...

So, in MiMi's Cafe I drink my mocha latte, let my children comfort me, and dry my eyes on my napkin.

Twenty-Eight

Dive

Edd is a gifted musician. He sings Steven Curtis Chapman songs beautifully. He'll sit with the honey-colored guitar on his lap and strum into the night, the music filling our house and spilling out to the silent forest. The words reflect our life:

> "What about the change
> What about the difference
> What about the grace
> What about forgiveness
> What about a life that's showing
> I'm undergoing
> the change."

Edd, the kids, and I go to a Steven Curtis Chapman concert in Anaheim. The Arrowhead Pond is a hockey rink for the Mighty Ducks. For events other than hockey, they cover the ice and put up a stage. The Pond is a huge enclosed dome. From our up-high seats, we feel like we are in a spaceship, looking down on the distant stage, surrounded by rows of people and lights.

Steven's concert theme is "God can turn sorrow to joy." He sings "When Love Takes You In," a tear-jerker about how he and his wife, even though they already had three children of their own, traveled all the way to China to adopt a baby girl who was abandoned by the side of the road.

A big screen shows videos of children and landscapes, so that we didn't just focus on the short man on the stage (If I ever talk to large groups, I wouldn't want them staring at my face all the time, but looking above me at photos of the natural world: mountains and trees and rocky ocean cliffs spreading toward sunset...).

A child's face speaks more than words. Something in the eyes tells us about God's love:

> "When love takes you in
> everything changes.
> A miracle starts
> with the beat of a heart
> And this love will never let you go."

Then he sings a song that speaks to my own unanswered sorrows:

> "And the pain falls like a curtain
> On the things I once called certain.
> And I have to say the words I fear the most;
> I just don't know.
>
> And the questions without answers
> Come and paralyze the dancer,
> So I stand here on the stage afraid to move.
> Afraid to fall, oh, but fall I must.
> On this truth that my life
> has been formed from the dust.
>
> God is God and I am not.
> I can only see a part
> of the picture He's painting.
> God is God and I am man;
> So I'll never understand it all,
> For only God is God."

"Let God write the story of your life," Chapman says when he ends the song. "It may not make sense now, but the story is not finished."

Chapman then turns to his left to welcome a friend. A man named Steve Saint walks on stage. He is the son of Nate Saint, one of five missionaries killed in the Amazon jungle in 1956. They had brought their wives and young children with them to the verge of the rainforest, a land of thick trees and rivers, bright flowers and rainbow-colored birds. The men then left camp and flew in a yellow airplane to the edge of a river deep inside the impassible trees. They made contact with the warlike Auca Indians and even took amateur movies of partially-clad natives examining their plane and running along the river, holding up a yellow toy model airplane that soared through the thick moist air.

A few days later the anxious wives at Base Camp lost radio contact with their husbands, and within a week all five bodies were found floating in the river not far from their speared-up plane.

Steve Saint was five years old.

One of the other missionaries who was killed left three children. Before he went on his last flight, he wrote in his journal:

"He is no fool who gives what he cannot keep to gain what he cannot lose."

His name was Jim Elliot. His widow, Elizabeth, wrote a famous little book about the whole ordeal. It's called Through Gates of Splendor.

But the story doesn't stop there. Steve Saint tells us about a movie coming out soon that finishes the tale. It's called Beyond the Gates. It tells how Nate Saint's sister went to live with the Aucas and spent the rest of her life winning their friendship and translating the Bible into their language. When she died of cancer, she was buried in the jungle not far from where her brother was killed.

And one of the men who helped spear Steve Saint's father to death befriended Steve when Steve came to visit his aunt.

That man, named Mincaye, became "Grandfather" to Steve's children and a leader in the ever-growing church among the Amazon indians.

As Steve tells us this, Mincaye comes on stage. Mincaye speaks to the audience in his own language, translated by Steve.

"I am a God-follower," Mincaye says. "And you all should go and tell your friends as my people travel through the jungle to tell our neighbors. We speak the news that God sent His son to walk our trail with us and die and rise again so that death would not be our final home. We can go up to God's Big House and live forever—all part of one family."

The short, chubby, wide-footed man with dark skin and a feather crown on his head stands next to the tall, thin, blondish man in glasses and a white-collared shirt. Silence surrounds us in the huge round auditorium, holding us all for a moment. We are caught up in the same story—whether we are Indian or white or Asian or black or whatever—because that story is a variation of our own. God has sought each one of us, drawing us into a family that transcends the borders of time or race or religion or gender or nationality or city or island or mountain or rainforest.

Then Steve Saint turns to the audience and says,

"A fairy tale is not a fairy tale until the last chapter."

And I think, yeah. That is my story. How can I know the ending until I stand there and look back on the pattern I could not clearly see during its weaving?

Steven Curtis Chapman ends his concert with my favorite song, "Dive."

> "The long-awaited rains
> Have fallen hard upon the thirsty ground
> And carved their way to where
> The wild and rushing river can be found.
> And like the rains
> I have been carried here
> to where the river flows, yeah.

My heart is racing and my knees are weak
As I walk to the edge
I know there is no turning back
Once my feet have left the ledge.
And in the rush I hear a voice
That's telling me it's time
to take the leap of faith,
So here I go.

I'm diving in, I'm going deep
In over my head I want to be
Caught in the rush, lost in the flow,
In over my head I want to go.
The river's deep, the river's wide,
The river's water is alive.

So sink or swim, I'm diving in.

There is a supernatural power
In this mighty river's flow.
It can bring the dead to life,
And it can fill an empty soul
And give a heart the only thing
Worth living and worth dying for, yeah.

But we will never know the awesome power
Of the grace of God
Until we let ourselves get swept away
Into this holy flood.
So if you'll take my hand,
We'll close our eyes and count to three
And take the leap of faith.

Come on; let's go!"

 The words surround me. They create images in my mind. I am transported to the mountain forest. It is dry from drought.

Pine trees are turning brown and dying. Dust kicks up from my feet. I wander toward the Summit: bare and windswept and covered with white rock. And then, around a bend, I find the River. It rushes beneath the cliff I stand on: loud and swift and frightening. I push my toes to the edge and look down.

This is my life. I must not hesitate. I must dive.

My feet leave the rock, and for a moment I fall through the air. Then my hands and head break through the water. It is alive. My body plunges through it. Bubbles and currents surround me as I stroke deeper.

God is not someone we tolerate for an hour on Sunday. His book is not a boring history lesson. His words are love letters eagerly devoured—water for the thirsty—rivers beyond measure, oceans deeper than we can imagine:

> "O God, You are my God;
> early will I seek You;
> my soul thirsts for You;
> my flesh longs for You
> in a dry and thirsty land
> where there is no water." (Psalm 63:1)

> As the deer pants
> for the water brooks,
> so pants my soul for You, O God.

> My soul thirst for God,
> for the living God.
> When shall I come and appear
> before God?

> My tears have been my food
> day and night,
> while they continuously say to me,
> 'Where is your God?'

O my God, my soul is cast down within me;
therefore I will remember You
from the land of the Jordan,
and from the heights of Hermon,
from the Hill Mizar.

Deep calls unto deep
at the noise of Your waterfalls;
all Your waves and billows
have gone over me." (from Psalm 42)

I have never been to Israel. I have never stood in the Jordan River where John baptized Jesus. I have never climbed Mount Hermon to the northeast, where once the Cedars of Lebanon stood. But I know what a dry land is, and I have flown in a helicopter to the Wettest Spot on Earth.

God's river is like the crater of Mount Waialele in Kauai, where clouds always cover the summit, and waterfalls cascade down thousands of feet in a perfect circle.

"But whoever drinks of the water
that I shall give him
will never thirst.
But the water
that I shall give him
will become in him
a fountain of water
springing up into everlasting life." (John 4:14)

God can heal whatever hurts us. Don't wait on the dry ledge. Dive into the river. Stand inside the waterfall.

Twenty-Nine

Pink Badge of Courage

Autumn is here again.

In the mountains, the deciduous trees change colors. Their brilliant red, pink, orange, and yellow leaves contrast with the tall evergreens, silver rocks, and blue sky. The wind blows through everything.

I love the wind. I open the housedoors and windows and say,

"Come in! Clean out all the dust and cobwebs!"

Jesus said:

"The wind blows where it wishes,
and you hear the sound of it,
but cannot tell where it comes from
and where it goes.

So is everyone who is born
of the Spirit." (John 3:8)

Last October, after my fifth miscarriage, I prayed desperately that by this same time next year the whole baby thing would be resolved—one way or another. I said this prayer for Cherie, too, and she got pregnant a few months later. She had a flawless pregnancy. Today, a year after my prayer, on October 10, Cherie easily delivered a perfect baby boy. She and her husband Bill named him Buck (to keep their tradition of

"B" names for all their children). Now Cherie can use that baby room and all those baby clothes and accessories she saved. Now she can walk around with a baby sling across her shoulder while everyone admires her little bundle. Now she can attach a fifth little silver magnetic fish, swimming after two big ones, to the back of her gigantic passenger van.

I realize that I sound a little sarcastic and bitter. I admit that those silver fish on the back of Cherie's van bug me—like trophies hung on a wall.

I feel like Laura Ingalls Wilder, the nineteenth-century writer of children's books. She grew up on the American prairie, in the time of pioneers and covered wagons. She married young and had a baby girl named Rose. Then she had a baby son who died. She and her husband put him in a little wood casket and stood vigil through the night. Her husband's crops failed, so they couldn't buy supplies. They barely survived a winter blizzard. Their house burned to the ground.

Laura and her husband decided to move to a new home, away from the prairie. They packed their few remaining belongings and their young daughter onto a wagon and said goodbye to Laura's family. Before they drove away, Laura turned to her father and said,

"I miss those childhood days when I felt safe inside our cabin, by the cheerful fire, as you played your fiddle, and Ma and we children danced. I thought that nothing could hurt me as long as you were there. Why didn't you tell me it would be so hard?"

Laura was sixty when she started writing her childhood stories. Though she was growing old, she wrote with the heart of a child, creating in simple words her prairie world of wind-blown grass, sudden clouds, and vast horizons. A publisher once told her to change her narration, to add sophistication and style and craft, but Laura kept her own voice, and her Little House on the Prairie books became children's classics.

I think, that to her dying day, Laura remembered that infant boy she buried on the prairie.

I find it ironic (so typical of my life) that on the same

day as Cherie had her baby boy, I drive down the mountain for the Light of Hope celebration at a Cancer Care Center. Edd stayed with the children (I invited Jessica for a mother-daughter bonding experience, but she didn't want to come. I can't blame her; she's only ten and doesn't want to think about the sisterhood of breast cancer survivors).

So I get an evening to myself, a rare event. I drive down the mountain at twilight. The crescent moon shines through wispy clouds as the last pastel lights of sunset silhouette the dark mountains. I push my Subaru to its limits, screeching around curves and leaving slow flatlanders behind. I laugh out loud at the rush, the windows down, the cool autumn air catching the sound and sending it up into the darkness.

I love black. My high school art teacher called it "the absence of color," but I disagree. It is a beautiful color. I almost always wear it, though Jessie declares (with a disapproving sigh, after looking through my closet), "Mom, you can't wear black forever." Black makes me look thinner. Black is elegant and rich and deep and mysterious. God made the night to contrast with a single point of light—like the first star above the mountain, the sole house on a distant ridge, a reflector square in the asphalt road, or a diamond against velvet. Black is serene, calm, uncomplicated, at rest.

But as I drive further down the mountain highway, I am heading toward a million lights in the vast valleys and cities of California. There are so many lights that they create a yellow haze, a layer I drive through like a cloud. Freeways weave together like glowing snakes as I approach the city's heart. Eighteen-wheel freight trucks surround me, heading for the Port and their waiting cargo. Shiny clean sports cars speed toward a night in Hollywood, their chrome and waxed metal hoods reflecting my headlights. I don't think my old Subaru, caked with mountain dust and pine needles, reflects much of anything...

As cars and trucks pass me, I feel the heartbeat of the city. Roads spread in all directions. Long trains clatter along on unseen tracks to my left. I pass the International Airport with its green threshold lights, red warning lights, and white runway markers. Jets lift off with strobelights and winglights flashing. I could go anywhere…

After driving for an hour and a half, I finally find the Cancer Care Center, not far from where I heard Carrie Fischer speak. It's a low, modern building with a large round fountain in front, in the middle of a circular tiled driveway. The fountain is surrounded by glowing paper bags, each with a single candle in it. The bags spill out toward the walkway and along the terra cotta building. I park the car and walk up the drive, taking photos of the lighted fountain. I walk inside and notice that the walls are painted various shades of pink. Even the floor has a peach-colored carpet. A greeter hands me a basket that holds pink ribbons. I pin one on my sparkly black tunic and take one for Gloria, my adopted Jewish mother who also survived breast cancer.

The Cancer Care Center director greets me (I sent her a copy of <u>Crossing the Chemo Room</u>, and she mailed me back an actual thank-you note). She shows me tables of catered food: chocolates, fruit, pastries, crackers, cheese, punch, champagne. I pick up some breast cancer pamphlets from another table and head to the Ladies Room, which is done all in pink tile.

I wander out to the lawn, where a white tent is set up, and listen to breast cancer survivors tell their stories. I sit at a round table covered with a pink tablecloth, with a pink glass jar in the middle that holds a candle. Another survivor sings a song. Volunteers hand out candles.

There are not just women here. I see men, children, old, young, all races, all colors, all beliefs…Cancer does not discriminate.

Someone reads a long list of names from a scroll: those who have survived cancer. I hear Gloria's name, and my own. Someone else reads a shorter list of those who died of the disease. We are all silent. The names hang in the night air like points of light.

A rustle of motion begins at the edge of our circle. People start passing flame from candlewick to candlewick until we all hold flames high against the dark autumn night. The candles illumine our faces. Some of us do not have any hair or eyebrows. But we all have eyes that reflect the fire, and we wear pink ribbons against our breasts—our symbol of survival.

Our scar, our wound of battle, our Pink Badge of Courage.

Thirty

The Morning Star

I come near the end of this book I didn't want to write, and I realize it is probably the best thing I will ever write. Yet how shall I finish? Can I tie up each event and emotion like neat pink ribbons made into a bow?

My life is like the contrast of beautiful Kauai and New York on September 11, 2001.

On September 11, Jessica asked "Why isn't it a good world?" and I tried to assure her that much of it still is.

If we look, we can find beauty around us. God made amazing things like mountains with summits of white rock above evergreen forests. In the mountains of Asia, above 10,000 feet, snow leopards hunt at night, moonlight glistening on their silvery coats.

Those coats made poachers hunt them to near extinction. Who could kill a leopard for its coat? Who could wear such a treasure, hang it on the wall, or hide it in a closet? Maybe someday we will see snow leopards only in museums—stuffed and silent and still—or as images on glowing computer screens. Our world is better for the few snow leopards left in the wild, prowling secretly in places humans could not survive.

In the North American mountains where I live are hawks and eagles. They pair-bond for life, but they unite with their mate only at breeding time, at the same nest year after year. They are mostly silent, solitary birds, content to soar alone on wind currents. These raptors work hard for their prey, diving

200 miles an hour to catch a mouse or rabbit. A hawk does not make an affectionate pet. If trained, it will merely tolerate its human as it would a familiar tree. It does not want to be petted. It perches silently on a leather glove, tethered, watching its surroundings with a hunter's eye.

People can be compared to snow leopards or hawks. Children, especially, are like an endangered species, more rare and precious than we imagine.

Selah explored many Zones as she climbed the Summit. Then she stood before a Portal and realized there are worlds out there that we cannot see, new dimensions, filled with colors beyond our spectrum.

We all stand between worlds, as if something like glass separates us from here and there.

When I had left the California city to live in the English countryside, I understood that separation one day when a muddy dog came up to my car and put his paws on my window:

"Blossoms"

"How far to the lodge?" I ask,
leaning out the window
of a rented car. An Englishman
in green Wellies and a wool cap
ambles toward me, a labrador frisking near.
I reach over glass and steel
for the narrow black head.
The dog does not wait for my hand;
she leaps, splattering mud
on window face and door,
on my forehead and pale sweater,
in the corner of my mouth.
I see the face of the Englishman,
the tongue and eyes of the dog,
and I want to kneel in three-inch muck,
embrace the lapping animal

until I'm covered with earth—
the gritty, tangy stuff I taste,
full of seeds, mingled with rainwater
and the prints of man and dog.
The person beside me moves the car in gear.
We pass slowly; I wipe off my arm,
roll up the window,
and see two brown marks
like blossoms
grown upon the glass.

Or it's like my raccoon story:

"Raccoons at Midnight"

The children and I hear strange noises that rouse us from our beds. We turn the light on outside the back deck and find a raccoon sitting on our woodpile. In the housecorner another bandit face stares at us, eyes reflecting the light.

We fetch cat food, open the sliding glass door, and offer the raccoons dinner. A mother comes out, followed by three babies. I shut the door again because they are wild creatures and could bite or scratch or make a mess in our house.

The raccoons are beautiful, their fur black and white, with a striped fluffy tail. They gather in a circle and use their long black paws like hands to scoop the cat food to their mouths. We take photos, and the flash doesn't scare them away. We watch, the glass between us in our heated den and these wild creatures on the cold deck. The dark forest, stars, and moon seem to swirl around them.

One brave baby raccoon puts his paws up on the glass, and Jonathan bends down to place his hands over them, the glass between their touching.

Later, he would type this poem on the computer, for the Homeschool Fair, where he won a Blue Ribbon:

"The Black Raccoon"

by Jonathan Williams

age 7

A black raccoon
lives under my deck
and in the night
she comes to me

with her black cubs
and their white tails
with bandit faces
and bright brown eyes

I feed them snacks
they use their paws
delicately
to eat the food

and when they're done
they look through the glass
curious

And Jessica won a Blue Ribbon for her close-up digital photo of Penny, the bright green and yellow Senegal parrot. Jessie caught Penny's profile, showing the sharp curved black beak with little gray feathers at the top. Penny's honey-colored eye held still with its dark pupil reflecting a single point of light.

I have always been drawn to the light. As a baby, I stared at glass prisms, silver ornaments—anything that glistened. When I was a child, sitting in the back of a police car while my mother and stepfather were being arrested for public drunkenness when we were living in a tent, I stared at the gold crucifix I held in my hands as sunlight shone through the squad car window onto it. And I realized that sunlight on gold was made by Someone wonderful, who loves me, who can make my life beautiful, too.

Even now, I like to wear crystals and watch the light shine through them into rainbows. Why should witches and New Agers only get to do that?

I, like Selah of the Summit, have escaped the darkness of witchcraft. In college, I knew a friend who wrote a book called <u>Escape from Witchcraft</u>. I used to hike in the forests where she and her coven had sacrificed animals and performed dark rituals. I would find bleached bones on stone altars. Now I can walk out on my deck in the moonlight, lift my arms above my head, and dance in the forest. The moon, nearly full, shines through the branches of the tall silver fir which grows above my house. Why should witches only enjoy the moon? I know the One who made it.

In Bolivia, in the mountains, lives a tribe of people who are all witches. They believe that each mountaintop has its own demon, and that they must be careful not to offend the devil who controls the earth. They are a violent people, often having fights or murders after they drink alcohol or use drugs. They carry around rat poison in case they meet an angry fellow witch. They would rather commit suicide than be beaten to death. When they enter a church, they feel relief from their constant physical pain. With empty eyes they stare at the speaker as God's words penetrate the darkness woven around them by witchcraft.

Even in ancient Israel, the prophets warned of the dangers of "the high places," where pagan altars were built and babies sacrificed to bloodthirsty gods.

But there are holy mountains. God gave Moses the Ten Commandments on Mount Sinai. Solomon built the Temple on Mount Zion in Jerusalem. The most amazing mountain was a hill in Jerusalem. It was called Golgotha, Place of the Skull, where Jesus was crucified. He shed His blood so that the mountain demons could not destroy us. And now, because of freedom in Him, we can enjoy the heights because God made them and has triumphed over "the prince of the power of the air, the spirit who now works in the sons of disobedience." (Ephesians 2:2)

And there was another mountain, where Peter saw Christ transfigured, glowing brighter than the sun:

> "For we did not follow cunningly devised fables
> when we made known to you
> the power and coming of our Lord Jesus Christ,
> but were eyewitnesses of His majesty.
>
> For He received from God the Father
> honor and glory
> when such a voice came to Him
> from the Excellent Glory:
> 'This is My beloved Son,
> in whom I am well pleased."
>
> And we heard this voice
> which came from heaven
> when we were with Him
> on the holy mountain.
>
> We also have the prophetic word made more sure,
> which you do well to heed
> as a light that shines in a dark place,
> until the day dawns
> and the morning star rises in your hearts." 2 Peter 1:14-19

Those last verses are so cool. Christ is a light shining in a dark place. Someday we will see Him face to face, as a new day dawns. And He, like the Morning Star, will rise in our hearts.

Selah journeyed from the hot, oppressive valley to the mountains. She climbed past deserts and hillsides, oakgroves and meadows, moors and cliffs, lakes and waterfalls, until she reached the Summit. There she stood on the highest spot. All around her mountains curved in blue-green layers, spreading in a circle, touching the horizon on every side.

Above the Summit spreads the azure sky, and at the very zenith stands a portal filled with stars...

> "And he carried me away in the Spirit
> to a great and high mountain,
> and showed me the great city,
> the holy Jerusalem,
> descending out of heaven from God.
>
> Having the glory of God.
> Her light was like a most precious stone,
> like a jasper stone,
> clear as crystal..." Revelation 21:10-11

Thirty-One

Christmas in Lothlorian

It's Christmas again. I burst into tears at random times: tears for baby Michael who died five years ago, tears for my father who shot himself when I was almost five, tears for my mother and my lost brother Kerry and the grandmother I remember.

Sometimes I walk along a lakeside trail at dusk and stare up at the stately houses that look more like hotels than homes. Their tall proud windows are dark and empty of light because their rich owners, who mostly live in the city, rarely visit the mountains. The houses have gables and decks and high, impressive doors. Their front yards sweep down among pine trees and sculptured hedges to private docks at the lakeshore.

I try to remember my grandmother's manorhouse, which she sold to strangers, and wonder if it is empty now.

Christmas is a stressful time. It brings out dormant sorrows and angers. It forces families together or apart, makes people confront things, causes contemplation of the passing year.

This Christmas, my niece Linda is living for the first time in a safe place away from her abusive family. She has been adopted by the Connelleys, old friends of ours from the valley. I ended <u>Crossing the Chemo Room</u> in Heidi's living room, where she was holding a women's Bible study and tea. Now Heidi, her husband, and her children live on a ranch with animals on a wide, rocky land beneath a clear sky. They have made room for Linda, who can take piano lessons and gather eggs from chickens and jump high on the backyard trampoline.

Chris also recently left his father to live with our old friend Marvin. Chris and Linda's father gave up his apartment and is living out of his car.

And there is another whose life was spared.

Chelsea Smith, the teenager who spent the entire summer in a hospital, fighting Crohn's disease, stood beside her father this Christmas and sang the opening solo for the Twentieth Annual Singing Christmas Tree. She stood like a princess in a black velvet tunic, her golden hair curling around her shoulders. She smiled, her cheeks chubby from Prednisone, her eyes glittering in the spotlight.

I couldn't stop the tears from running down my face as she sang, and I remembered those days in the hospital when we visited her, bringing presents or crafts. I remembered her artwork that Chelsea decorated the walls with—flowers in pastel pinks and blues and yellows, painted on wooden plaques and boxes, entwined with green leaves. And the I.V lines running into her thin arms and the bruise marks from needles, and knowing she was bleeding internally and couldn't even drink water. And we brushed her long hair and gave her a glowing crystal necklace so that she looked like a princess, small and frail...

Steve's clear tenor voice brought me back to the present, as he joined in a duet with the daughter he could have lost. He smiled, his Santa Claus cheeks rosy above his graying beard and his eyes bright behind his gold-rimmed glasses. The light caught his black tuxedo and green waistcoat, mixing colors with the clear notes of music that sang to the Christchild:

"Welcome to our world."

And Edd's face also ran with tears, and surely anyone in the audience who knew the Smith's story could not help but feel awe—like a spring bubbling up within them—as they witnessed this Christmas miracle.

This Christmas we traveled to Arizona. We visited my half-brother Bob who found me two years ago. He took us horseback riding in the red rock hills and introduced us to his children and granddaughter (who is only 3 years younger than Jonathan).

Bob's wife Sandy made us big pasta meals around a large table, and her grown-up children Dustin and Robin taught Jonathan how to play poker (which he is very good at). We had a lot of fun, but Bob and I got into arguments late at night, standing in a doorway at his house.

Bob focuses on the suffering in this world and blames God. He grew up without a good father figure, since our alcoholic dad left him before he left me (on the day he killed himself when I was nearly five years old). Bob became a Chicago police officer, so you can imagine that he saw a lot of bad things happen.

"But can't you see the beauty in the world?" I asked, my words like a silver sword held poised above me. "And can't you see that someday suffering will end because Christ came to bear the Curse and bring us new life? That's the meaning of Christmas: joy for all the people, as the angel said. Suffering will lie in the past, gone, forgotten, like stepping through a doorway, from one side to the other..."

"God is a sadist," Bob retorted, and I felt the anger in him as he raised his words like a broad black sword to slam against mine. Edd, as big as Bob and more intimidating with his full red beard and broad shoulders, walked over to us. His blue-green eyes frowned under their bushy brows, urging me to silence.

"Don't argue," Edd said in a low voice. "You will not change Bob's view. People see what they want to see."

When we returned to the hotel room, I felt the exhaustion of battle—and wished that my brother Bob would become a spiritual brother, too.

It was nice to get back to our mountain. I live in a place like Lothlorian, forest home of Elves. My house is wood, tall like a fortress, built among the trees that tower over it in tiers of graceful branches. At Christmastime, we place small white lights among the wood and greenery, like Galadriel's kingdom glowing with lanterns. Music resounds from our house, filling the forest with voices and stringed instruments.

I sit at my bedroom window and watch the sun shine on new snow which covers the slope and streambed. The snow weighs down the evergreens, making different patterns on different types of leaves. It is almost too bright for my eyes.

One of my favorite things to do is to fall straight back into new snow (you need a good foot or two) and lie there, upheld as if by faith. When I first did this in front of Jessica and Jonathan, they laughed at their silly mother.

I imagine lying in the snow as sunlight slants across the field of white and shines into my window. The sunbeam lights up my glass oil lamp that Edd gave me on our anniversary—and crystal vase filled with yellow silk daffodils that Dr. Schinke's office gave me when I finished my chemo treatments. The sunlight dances upon the gold candle snuffer and a big silver key.

"What is that key to?" my children once asked me, imagining a huge door with a keyhole so large.

"To my castle in England," I replied. They quietly accepted my words.

But now I think it is to my castle here, in the California mountains, in my place like Lothlorian.

And when the moon rises, I will stand at the edge of a mountain lake and watch the colors change in the sky above the dark treeline. Pink will melt to green and yellow and blue. The water will light up with the moon's reflection, ever changing on the waves, and a voice will whisper,

"He who made this
can do anything."

Toward midnight, I will rise from sleep and stare out my window. The moon will shine upon the new snow of the forest, contrasting white with the shadows of trees.

And, like Galadriel—wise and beautiful and fading from this world, Queen of the Elves, and keeper of a ring of power—I will know that a dark force encroaches from the lands below. But I will not wait for it to come. I will follow Aragorn and his keen sword. We will go to the darkest places where slaves are chained behind thick stone doors. We will bring a little light and tell about the mountains.

Edd, who looks like Aragorn when he wears his black

hooded cape and golden sword, takes me to see The Two Towers. It is a long, exhausting battle, with changes from the book and new characters. I like The Fellowship of the Ring better because of the different lands and the Elves—and, of course, Lothlorian.

But The Two Towers is good. The New Zealand scenery reveals the new land of Rohan, rolling red hills below snow-covered mountain ranges. Rohan is where the horsemen ride, men of long blonde hair and helmets. Edheras is their walled city on a hill beneath those mountains, its wooden buildings carved and painted like the old Viking villages.

The character of Eowyn is interesting. She steps out onto a stone step high atop Edheras, in front of the Great Hall. The constant wind blows her blonde hair across her face, and the flag of Rohan, a prancing white horse against a field of black, breaks free from its pole and lands at the approaching steps of Aragorn—a symbol for the returning king of Middle-earth.

Aragorn has ridden with Legolas, Gimli, and Gandalf to help defend Rohan. Eowyn sees him and is glad. She is a warrior princess who can wield a sword and would rather fight than flee with the other women.

Her uncle, Theodin, King of Rohan, is also interesting. At first he appears as a feeble old man under someone else's control. When Gandalf enters the cold Hall of the King, he confronts the King's assistant, Grima Wormtongue, who is Saruman's henchman. When Grima tries to stop Gandalf, Gandalf raises his white carved staff and says,

"I have not passed through death and fire to bandy words with a witless worm!"

And he delivers Theodin from Saruman's evil possession. Then King Theodin regains his strength. But he is torn between retreat and fighting. He wants to protect his people, so he flees with them to Helms Deep, a fortress cut into the mountains. Once there, he is unsure of the path ahead, though Aragorn urges him to go out and meet the enemy. King Theodin struts around the castle walls, ranting like a Shakespearean character:

"Who am I?"

"Is this the price that we must pay?"

"Then let them come."

After doing his best to defend his people against the orc hordes and Saruman's power, King Theodin finally goes on the offensive and rides out to meet his enemy. Clothed in gilded armor and atop a fine horse, Theodin finds his heroic role at last.

But, near the end of the movie, Sam becomes a more humble hero. The chubby little hobbit from The Shire, the gardener who never wanted to leave his home, who straps pots and pans on his back and tries to keep Frodo from the clutches of The Ring, saves Frodo's life. The Ring has become heavier and more enslaving the closer it gets to Mordor and its Master. Several times it has tried to destroy Frodo until it leads him to a crumbling tower of Gondor during a battle. Frodo, swaying on his feet, stands before a ringwraith riding a dragon.

Sam sees what is happening and tackles his friend before the beast can grab him in its talons. Frodo falls down the steps and then draws his sword Sting, thinking Sam wants to take away the precious Ring. But Sam tells Frodo, "It's only me. It's only your Sam."

Frodo pauses a moment, the glistening sword still held to Sam's bare throat.

Then he lays the sword down, weeping. Sam clasps his weary friend's hand and says, in a voice thick with the country accent of The Shire,

"In all the great stories, the ones that really matter, there were dangers and difficulties. Folk in those stories had plenty of chances to turn back. But they didn't."

"Why?" Frodo asks.

"Because they knew there was something worth fighting for in the world."

Later, as the two hobbits journey back toward Mordor, Sam says,

"I wonder if folk will weave a tale about us. 'That Frodo, wasn't he brave? Tell me again about Frodo and The Ring.'"

Frodo laughs, adding,

"I couldn't have done this without you, Sam. They'll talk about Sam the Wise too."

And so the hobbits travel on, Gollum always nearby to help or to betray. In the distance the smoking mountain of Doom rises into a red sky.

As Edd and I leave that theater, walking down a dark stairwell toward the exit, I think, I will never write a story as good as The Lord of the Rings.

> Then I realize,
> there are stories,
> there are great stories,
> and there is The Greatest Story Ever Told—
> and I am part of that.

Thirty-Two

The publishing world is a Tower guarded by the Dark Lord

It's a New Year. Possibilities abound.

We're on a vacation: down the mountain, past the hot valleys and sprawling cities, to the coast. We stay at a resort on an ocean bluff. The grounds are landscaped with fern trees, date palms, and Bird of Paradise flowers. We swim in a pool, baste in a jacuzzi, or walk along the seashore. The place reminds me of Kauai, with the fresh salt breeze and sound of crashing waves.

While doing bead crafts at the Activity Center, we meet a family from New Zealand.

Jonathan announces, "I look like Frodo, and I'm going to be an actor when I grow up."

Jessie says, "I want to move to New Zealand and live on a sheep farm."

The two New Zealand girls (the same age as my children) silently watch my brash Americans. Liz, the New Zealand mom, smiles and offers to give us a tour if we end up in Wellington.

"Someone my husband works with knows Peter Jackson," she tells us, and I imagine that every other New Zealander knows the famous director of <u>The Lord of the Rings</u>.

David, who is nineteen and has spiked black hair, works at the Activity Desk. He brings us more multi-colored beads to assemble. He has become the surrogate big brother for Jess and Jon this week while Ryan works at his auto mechanic shop.

David joins in our discussion about the making of <u>The Lord of the Rings</u>.

"That was a cool movie," he says. "Beautiful scenery and great sword shots."

"Did you know they tore down most of those lovely sets?" Liz informs us. "They should have left them there for the tourists."

"Yeah," I agree, wishing we could have walked through the carved white archways of Rivendell or climbed the treehouses of Lothlorian.

David lets me use the Activity Desk phone when an editor from Harcourt Brace publishers calls me back (I found their phone number on the Internet; it was unlisted in the phone book). An editor named Heidi tells me I can drive down to San Diego and drop off my books for her to look at. After hanging up the phone, I tell David the good news. He congratulates me with a high-five handshake.

I take the kids with me on the drive because Edd wants to rest in the hotel room. We navigate through unfamiliar traffic to the skyscrapers of downtown San Diego. I turn the excursion into a field trip, pointing out familiar landmarks amidst the unfamiliar new buildings going up everywhere.

"Oooh, there's a building that looks like the tower of Saruman at Isengard," Jessica says, pointing to the sharp white steeples of the new Mormon Temple, a building thrusting up toward heaven.

"There's Mission Bay and Sea World, and there's Mission Valley and Old Town," I say as we drive further south.

"Can you believe that Kristen and Ryan grew up here?" Jessie asks, amazed at the roads and houses everywhere.

We follow the directions the receptionist at Harcourt gave us, passing one-way streets at the foot of forty-storey buildings. We park in the garage of the Golden Eagle Building, emerge, and stare up at the glass and concrete structure. In the afternoon sunlight it looks like a castle or a fortress—not easily entered. I think of the Dark Lord's Tower in Mordor, guarded with a spiked metal gate. Jess gives Jonathan a piggyback ride into the elevator. He's wearing his binoculars so that he can "watch people," and several businessmen in black suits stare at us. We press a backlit brass button and shoot swiftly to the Nineteenth Floor.

We find the friendly receptionist. I write a note to Heidi the editor and leave my books with a business card. The receptionist calls the editor to say that I'm here, but Heidi explains she's too busy to meet me. She will pick up the books later.

Little do I realize that by the time I get home from vacation, I'll find a generic letter from Harcourt, saying they don't accept unsolicited manuscripts. Heidi didn't even look at my books that I hand-delivered, with two children as my escorts. She could have been honest with me and saved me the trip. Where is that door, opening?

> The publishing world is a Tower
> guarded by the Dark Lord.
>
> If you can't get in
> through the Big Black Gate,
> Like Frodo,
> Find another way.

Maybe I'm supposed to stay with GreatUnpublished.com, a young, high-tech, on-demand publisher. Maybe I'm supposed to be part of that publishing revolution.

Still, I feel depressed at the lack of actual money. Well, that's why God made tea and chocolate—to help me through disappointments. Of course, some things even tea and chocolate can't help, and that's when I need to go into the forest, sit under a tree, and pray.

At least my family encourages me. Edd prays for me and my books. When I get something published, he says "it's well deserved." He takes me to a local coffee house and plays Steven Curtis Chapman music, his guitar ringing loud and joyful (Edd could have been a lounge singer). He writes songs for me, putting his poetry to good use and helping me believe anything can happen.

Kristen and Ryan tell me they always liked the stories I told them when they were little.

I read <u>Selah</u> to Jessica and Jonathan at bedtime. I sit on Jonathan's bed, and he snuggles up to me. I embrace his slender shoulders and smell his curly hair, all while he fidgets and breathes and hums within the circle of my arms. I feel safe and comforted here with him, hidden in the mountains, away from the commercial publishing world.

Across from me, Jessie sits up on her bed. The children's bright eyes watch me in the dim light of a flashlight as I wrap them in my words:

One night, as Selah expected, Regan returned to confront her as she sat on her cot, resting. This time he brought her a silver tray covered with fresh fruit and cakes, with a bottle of wine next to two crystal chalices. He set the tray down on the wooden table. He did not yell as she expected but spoke in a quiet voice that was almost kind:

"You have been eating bread and water for several weeks now, so I thought you might want something tastier."

He opened the wine bottle and poured the red liquid into the chalice. Then he handed her a small white cake decorated with frosted rosebuds.

Regan did this all so naturally that Selah started to reach out her hand toward him. He smiled at her, and once again she noticed the glittering white of his teeth and the pale bluish-gray of his eyes.

A vision of Micah's red hair and deep blue eyes appeared between her and Regan. Selah withdrew her hand and hid it under her cloak, amazed that she had been so close to accepting a gift from her enemy.

Regan's eyes blinked, and for a moment he stopped smiling. Then he continued his ruse, pouring wine into the other chalice. "If you do not feel like drinking this fine wine, then I will," he said, lifting the red-filled cup to his pale lips. Selah watched, fascinated despite herself. Then a vision of the child with golden-red hair and blue-green eyes made her look away.

"I will not drink with you," she said, getting up from the cot and moving toward the far wall. "When will you let me leave this place and return to the Summit?"

Regan stared at her. He raised one eyebrow, amazed that Selah still had hope.

"Never," he replied. "You might as well accept that fact."

He watched his words sink into her mind. Selah's green eyes glazed over like the dead bird's.

"You don't have to stay in this small, hot room, you know," he continued slowly. "My own quarters are large and airy, with open windows and fans blowing cool air through them. You could walk freely through my suite and enter the Hexagon Room where secrets you cannot imagine wait for your discovery. You could have the whole Keep to explore, and even the gardens around it. You could wear robes of scarlet and gold instead of that homespun wool cloak that you refuse to remove even in this heat."

Selah said nothing. She stood with her back to the wall, trying to remember what it felt like to stand on the edge of a cliff in the rain, Micah beside her and the cool wind blowing her hair and cloak behind her like wings. She wished she had wings now so that she could fly away to the mountains.

Regan watched her for awhile, drinking the wine slowly.

"You are missing the delight of this good wine," he said after a while. Despite herself, Selah licked her lips. She wanted to taste the wine and the pretty white cakes decorated with rosebuds.

"I'm not as bad as you imagine," Regan continued, noticing the melting in Selah's resolve. "I can be very kind to those who are my friends. You don't need to fear me. See, I will put the tray at the end of the cot so that you don't have to come near me."

He placed the silver tray on the cot's edge. It glinted in the torchlight.

Selah tried not to stare at the tray. She looked at the floor, at the wall, at the torchlight. But her eyes were drawn toward the tray and what it held.

Selah was tired of bread and water—and even old cheese and dried dates from her traveling bag. The room felt so hot... Before she could talk herself out of it, she made one swift lunge for the tray, picked it up, and returned to her corner.

Regan smiled. Selah almost set the tray back on the cot, but something in Regan's smile made her hesitate. She reached one hand out to the crystal chalice. It felt smooth to her touch. She ran one finger around the circular top of the chalice. Before she quite realized what she was doing, she picked up the chalice and tasted the wine.

"I see you have some good sense. From now on, instead of bread and water, you will receive cake and wine each day." Regan stepped toward her, and Selah felt her strength melt slowly like ice in the warm room.

"I have something else for you," Regan said, holding out his arm, and a golden gown embroidered with red silk draped down toward the floor. Selah stared at it. Regan stepped toward her again. In his hand he held a gold tiara with a ruby center. "Let me put this on your head," he said, his words barely above a whisper. "It is The Crown of Celestia, brought down from the stars. It will turn you into a queen—and teach you many things. Exchange your shadowy hood for this crown. Take off your wool cloak and wear this lovely gown."

He stepped toward her.

Selah felt the heat surround her, and she longed to take off her cloak. The ruby in the gold tiara gleamed like power. Its deep red color made her remember all the scars she had received as a slave, all of the utter helplessness she had felt beneath the charge of someone else. Even on the journey to the Summit, she had been little more than baggage—following someone else's lead, under someone else's control.

Suddenly Selah wondered what it would be like to rule others. Perhaps if she wore The Crown of Celestia, she could rule even Regan...

"Take off your silver pendant and give it to me," Regan commanded quietly.

Selah put one hand on her silver pendant. It felt cold against her fingers, and she realized what Regan was trying to do.

"You are weaving The Craft on me," Selah accused, setting the crystal chalice down on the tray. "You are lying to me. You are trying to control me. You put something in the wine!"

Regan denied nothing.

"Stop fighting me, Selah. Surrender is easy. Here, try one of these."

He reached down, picked up a cake, and held it toward her.

"No," Selah replied quietly, folding her arms in front of her. "I will have no more of your Craft."

"Oh yes you will," Regan snarled, his eyes flashing with gray light. He raised his arm, and Selah found herself standing on a cliff, her feet at the very edge. She could not help but look downward. Flames licked up toward her from the smoky, unseen bottom. Curled fingers of red and black grabbed at her face and hair.

Terror like she had never known slashed through her body. Her legs felt weak. She could not catch her breath.

"This is the bottom of the crevasse, where Micah fell," Regan's voice bellowed from behind her. She could not turn around to face him.

"This is where you will go if you do not surrender."

Selah's head ached with the heat, and her vision started blurring. She felt her legs begin to buckle beneath her, but she could not scream or cry out for help. Her voice was frozen inside her.

Somehow she managed to move her left arm. Slowly she reached for her silver pendant. Her fingers closed around the cool metal, and strength returned to her legs. She turned to face Regan, holding up the pendant until it flashed coldly in the torchlight. She was back in her stone prison.

The first thing her eyes focused on was Regan's crystal sword, its tip held close to her chest. Selah was afraid to breathe, but she slipped her right hand into her traveling bag, brought out the silver dagger, and held it in front of her, tip to tip with Regan's sword. Regan stood firm. With one hand he fingered the white-gold triangles around his neck; with the other he held the sword in front of him. He spoke words Selah did not understand.

"You do not know what you are refusing," he said as if he had not just transported her to the edge of a fiery cliff. "I do not ask any slavegirl to be my Consort. Next time, I will not ask you. I will take what I want."

Selah stared at Regan, at his unblinking silver eyes, and she realized that his greatest weakness was his fierce pride. He thought he could not lose the battle. He had no idea what it was like to serve others—willingly—instead of control them.

"You cannot take me," Selah replied. "Or you would have done so already. The Maker will deliver me from you. He has given me a choice, and I have decided to serve Him."

At mention of the Maker, Regan winced as if in pain. He lowered his sword, pulled his silver cloak tightly around himself, turned, and left the room. Selah heard the door click locked behind him.

She stared at the crystal chalice still standing on the tray at the edge of her cot. The wine inside it looked like blood. She picked it up and threw it against the stone wall. It shattered into pieces and splattered the wine into a pattern she could not recognize. She then picked up the tray—cakes, fruit, and all—and flung it against the wall. It clattered to the stone floor with a ringing sound like music.

That gave Selah an idea. She grabbed her traveling bag and pulled out the silver flute. Without hesitating, she put the flute to her lips and blew. One long, high note filled the room, echoing against the stone walls.

Selah put the flute back in her traveling bag, sat down on the cot, and waited.

I finish the exciting part, mark the place with a piece of paper, and close the book. I can't fight back the tears that come to my eyes as I realize,

God, you have made me face my worst fears. People who read <u>Selah</u> will know that I lived this, that nonfiction blends with fiction in my life.

Before I can feel too sorry for myself, Jonathan solemnly pronounces:

"That's better than <u>The Lord of the Rings</u>."
"I wasn't in my bed anymore," Jessica adds.
And I realize,
maybe I am a writer...

I dream of places I've visited. I imagine people around me, like a giant network of life, and realize again how connected we are in this world...from my cousin's friend who worked at the World Trade Center in New York, to David at the Activity Desk by the sea, to the dark-skinned Hula dancers of Kauai, to the New Zealand family and their two shy girls with bobbed hair and names like Olivia, who come all the way across the Pacific, beneath the equator, from a land surrounded by oceans and covered with river gorges and snowy mountains and fantasy stories.

A door can open at any time. One minute my life can be going along in the same old exhausting, boring routine, and the next minute I can be flying off to New Zealand...

I wake up and watch Edd sleep for awhile, then rise and stare out my bedroom window. How bright and close the stars glow in the clear sky above the evergreen forest! I haven't seen stars for two weeks, since they were hidden by the Marine Layer at the beach.

I go to the bathroom for a drink. Even the tap water, drawn from our mountain lake, tastes cold and clean, unlike the tepid liquid of the lowlands.

Wherever I travel, I will belong at 6,000 feet.

And if the publishing world is a Tower guarded by the Dark Lord, at least I get to live on a mountain...

Thirty-Three

Witnesses

It's springtime again. I've been watching specials about the Holocaust on television. I cried when they showed the brave Jewish partisans who resisted Hitler during World War II. In a mountain forest below Russia, 1200 Jews were hidden in a makeshift town. They had their own shops, made their own food, and escaped the Nazis.

Another show was about Elie Weisel, a Nobel Peace Prize winner for literature. He is a Jewish writer and journalist who survived a concentration camp in World War II. As the television beamed black and white photos from the war, Elie's voice declared,

"God said to Israel long ago, 'You are my witnesses.' A witness has a special authority that cannot be questioned. I witnessed a great event in history, and I am duty-bound to tell about it."

Surely that command applies to me. I have witnessed strange and amazing things and must tell about them.

After Jesus rose from the dead, He called his disciples "my witnesses" and sent them out to spread Good News.

C.S. Lewis was another witness. He went from being an atheist to a Christian who could not help but write and speak about Christ.

On another T.V. night, I sat on the sofa and watched a man named David Payne play C.S. Lewis on stage. With a simple chair and a table set for tea, the chubby, middle-aged actor portrayed Lewis as if the audience were old friends, sitting in his study, chatting. I almost turned the show off and went to bed, for it had been a long day filled with housework and laundry. But something in the simple words stopped me.

Lewis told about his early years at Oxford, when he was walking with his friend Tollers (J.R.R. Tolkien) one night and discussing the idea of myth:

"'Isn't Christianity just another myth?' I asked Tollers. He paused for a moment in the half-light of the evening, turned to me, and said,

'No. This myth is Real, made by God Himself, who came to live among us.' It was late by then, and Tollers had to go home. But I stayed up, thinking about his words..."

And before Lewis quite realized what was happening, he became a Christian.

Lewis went on to talk about his alcoholic brother and his single life as an Oxford professor and his many books. I felt resentment toward him at that point. My writing life has never been as easy as one of those Oxford professors. For me, writing is pain—not only physical, of aching shoulders and neck and head from bending down to look at a computer screen and tired fingers from typing—but emotional and spiritual from pouring so much of myself into the words. And always come the interruptions and the countless other tasks...

Sometimes I want nothing more than a cruise to Alaska, with no computer or phone or emails, and a camera along only for fun.

I was really considering going to bed when Lewis started talking about the romance he found in his sixties, when he met Joy, the American divorcee who would become his wife. At first, he married her so that she and her young sons would not be deported from England. Then the doctors informed him that she had terminal bone cancer. They fell in love, and Lewis married her a second time for real.

"I never thought that in my sixties I'd find the Joy I missed in my twenties," Lewis said with a wink. "When she died, she smiled three times: first at the chaplain, then at me, and then...then at the Christ she could finally see. And her dying face reflected the glory of the Lord. The Bright and Morning Star shone upon her."

I was weeping at that point, grabbing tissues while Edd, making a snack in the kitchen, watched me curiously.

"Of course, I was angry and bitter about her death," Lewis continued as he poured a cup of tea. "My brother, who had come to love her as the sister we never had, did what he always did in a crisis. He turned to drink." He picked up a floral teacup and stared at the audience for a moment.

"But I...I picked up my pen and began to write."

And so was born the books <u>A Grief Observed</u> and <u>The Problem of Pain</u>.

Lewis continued: "I kept asking how could God do this? Then I realized I saw what we hadn't had, not what we had. When she got better after our real marriage ceremony, we expected at the most a few months. We got three years. She was my Gift. God was the Giver."

I felt, at that moment, that C.S. Lewis was my brother.

If Tolkien hadn't seen the horrors of World War I trench warfare, chemical weapons, airplane bombers, and fiery tanks, he couldn't have written about the evil Sauron in his burning Mount Doom. If Tolkien had not seen the Industrial revolution encroach on green English hillsides and forests, he could not have shown the fragile nature of The Shire. If Elie Weisel had not survived a concentration camp, he could not have written words that bring awareness to generations.

Springtime is always so busy. We celebrate Passover and Easter, start wrapping up the homeschool year, and go on field trips because the snow has finally left the mountains and we can drive safely:

"The Last Hayride"

Doris Bowers has been teaching her homeschool science

classes again. We missed the first two and were late to the last three. I can't get my act together before noon.

Doris' final class was about Birds. She held it at a ranch down in the valley, an hour's drive one way. We had to attend that class, even though none of us were feeling up to it. We got there after the lunch break, and I could tell by Doris' look that she was disappointed we missed her morning lecture.

I wondered if "better late than never" was true as I mumbled our excuse (though true) about Jessica's recent stomach problems, Jonathan's allergies, and my constant neuropathy.

It was a perfect day for birding—overcast and cool. Our homeschool group of various-aged children, mothers, and a couple of fathers, took a walk in search of nests. A mother red-tailed hawk and her mate had built a huge nest of sticks in the top of a tall eucalyptus tree, back against a canyon. When she spied us coming, she flew away, circling at a distance, watching us. When we walked under the nest, we could hear the babies calling.

We found an oriole's neat straw nest under a spreading palm branch, safe from heat and rain. We saw a swallow's mud nest on a building, up near the roof. We spied an owl hiding in the daylight, barely visible in oak branches.

Back at the classroom, Doris said a prayer to dismiss the class. After the other homeschoolers went home, the kids and I wandered about the room, looking at things we had missed: stuffed birds of prey with their wings spread wide, different types of eggs, feather collections, bird anatomy diagrams, photos, books. We decided to stay for a horseback ride and dinner, with a hayride to follow.

Dinner was in the ranch dining hall, at picnic-style tables with benches. The kids and I sat at the table with Doris, and she shared about her cancer.

"The sores on my leg are finally healing," she said, patting her right leg where the melanoma first appeared. "It used to ooze so much that no bandage worked. And I kept getting more brown patches."

I looked at her face, which was puffy from her last treatment. At least she had gained some weight, and her hair was thicker—white and wavy. But her left hand looked purplish and frail as she held her fork.

I hate what cancer does to people, I thought as I watched Doris eat with shaking hands.

But she still had her spunk. After dinner Doris organized the hayride, giving our small group instructions before we climbed onto the big trailer bed pulled by a tractor. The sun would set soon, and a cold wind blew down from the mountains where clouds gathered, dark and heavy.

The ranch manager, with his wife and little boy beside him, drove us across the highway to the neighbor's dairy farm. Cows ran to the fence, their black and white faces curious. We drove by irrigation channels newly wet with rain. The wind blew colder, and I huddled in my jacket and blanket, next to Christy.

Christy is twenty years old and responsible for her age. She has straight dark hair, impish brown eyes, and a playful smile. She grew up on a Christian camp in the mountains, on the far side by the wilderness, where I took Doris that day we saw egrets on a mountain lake. Christy, a natural teacher, is helping Doris with her classes and preparing to take them over.

Jonathan, further down the haystack row, chattered with some boys his age and played with his flashlight. Jessica, on the other side of me, leaned toward me and whispered,

"It's cold."

Doris, wearing her hat and gloves, stood up at the far end of the trailer and pointed to ducks on a little pond. All eyes followed her sweeping arm, then tried to focus with their binoculars. A few people checked their bird books. The sun dipped over the hills and painted the sky bright orange, and a few bright stars shone beneath the encroaching stormclouds.

We paused beneath a dark eucalyptus grove and made squeaky noises to lure out the owls. One glided silently from tree to tree, barely visible against the starlight. I thought I heard it call out softly, speaking Doris' name...Doris stood again and turned toward the sound, and I got the feeling she won't be doing many more hayrides. I imagined her sweeping up toward Heaven on a night like this, on a wagon of bird's wings, and sending down her coat to Christy—like Elijah threw his mantel from a fiery chariot, down to Elisha, the prophet of Israel who succeeded him.

Thirty-Four

Invitation

I am continuously amazed at the beauty of this world yet experience its suffering. I will dance with Edd, hike through the forest, and ice skate with my children. I will deal with the long-term effects of my disease and treatment, of the loss of my family, of the scars of miscarriages.

I know what it is to stand outside, in the dark, and look into a lighted window. I have watched a family sitting around their table that blazes with candlelight. The family laughs together, their honey-colored hair glowing with reflected light, their eyes alive with joy. I know what it is to wish I had a place at the table, with them, belonging, invited.

How many of us have been overlooked as a dinner guest? How many of us don't get asked to celebrations?

On top of the Summit a banquet table waits, with empty glass chairs in the snow near a frozen lake. The table stretches toward infinity, set with crystal goblets, etched silver, and china bordered by blue and gold. Each place setting is prepared, ready for anyone who answers the Invitation.

Jesus told the story about the king whose son was getting married. The king prepared his Great Hall with all types of food and entertainment. The king invited all his wealthy friends, but they were too busy with their own business. So he sent his servants out to the highways. They invited the poor, the forgotten, the diseased, the strangers—anyone who would come to the feast. (Matthew 22)

Why do we not answer the Invitation?

Perhaps we are too busy with our everyday lives.

Our Tax Man's wife Nancy died suddenly of a heart attack last Sunday night. No one expected it, though both Nancy and her husband George worked long, stressed hours preparing people's taxes. George was older and had more health problems, so everyone expected he would go first. They have one daughter, Elizabeth, who has young children and lives in Denver. How does Elizabeth feel now? Like I felt when my mother died suddenly on the other side of a continent, I got a phone call in the middle of the night, and I tasted nothing but ashes in my mouth.

Perhaps we think we don't need an Invitation.

Have you ever been lost in the forest? It's easier to do than you might think. I went for a hike with Jessica once, on the far side of the mountain, in the wilderness area where Christy, assistant to naturalist Doris Bowers, lives at a camp. We were unfamiliar with the terrain and hiked along a ridge, the Summit's white rock face always visible to our right. When we turned back, we could not find the camp. The day had been dry and hot, and all our water was gone. The sun was sinking behind the mountain. We had no compass, flashlight, or map. Our feet ached in their sturdy hiking boots. We stood, walking sticks in hand, and regarded a darkening forest with no visible paths. A long gorge dropped down to our left, filled with boulders, tree stumps, and shadow.

We finally found our way back to Christy's camp because we stumbled into a neighboring camp, and the owner guided us in the right direction.

One could say, how stupid to take a hike without proper preparation. But you cannot always tell where you will end up. Sometimes there are no maps. And if you stand in front of an unfamiliar forest and need to get through to the other side, wouldn't you rather have a Guide who knows the way—than depend on yourself, risk getting lost, and fall into an unseen crevasse?

On the night when Jesus celebrated His last Passover with

the disciples, after the meal, He wrapped a towel around his waist, took a bowl of water, and began washing His disciples' feet. Imagine their surprise as their Lord knelt before them and washed away dust and dirt, anointing them with water—a symbol of the Passover blood He would shed. (John 13)

He went to the grave and escaped into eternal life. What better Guide than that?

Perhaps we simply ignore the Invitation, offered to us by outstretched hands forever marked with red nail prints.

Our new church, Calvary Chapel, has a cool pastor named Tom. He's Italian, with warm brown eyes and olive-colored skin. He's always willing to give you a big hug, put his arms on your shoulder, and pray for whatever is bothering you. If you come at 10:30 on Sunday morning, you can get free coffee and muffins. One morning, as I reached for something to stir my French Vanilla coffee, I remarked,

"Cool. They've got toothpicks."

Then I realized I was pointing at popsicle sticks.

"Yeah, toothpicks for a dragon, maybe," Edd remarked, and we burst into laughter while Pastor Tom and his wife Sandi watched and wondered.

"I'm not a morning person," I explained. "Besides, I've been stuck in front of a computer screen too much lately. I'm losing my brain."

They agreed with me.

Our church sits atop the mountain. Its theme verse, written across the sanctuary in scrolling letters decorated with leaves and pine cones, says "I will bring them to my holy mountain and make them joyful in my house of prayer." (Isaiah 56:7)

You can stand on the edge of the churchyard and see a view of the whole mountain range—past forests, peaks, and lakes—to the wilderness, The Summit of nearly 12,000 feet, where I got lost once. Sometimes I go and stand at the edge, feel the wind blow over me, and say,

Thank you!

to my Guide through the Forest.

Our church had a banquet recently. The women decorated

the sanctuary with flowers and bows, tablecloths and centerpieces. They draped curtains on the walls and laid out silverware, handpainted china, and bowls of blue glass.

I wanted to invite all my friends. I wanted those with traumatic pasts, emotional problems, bad marriages, health conditions—any pain at all—to come to the feast so that we could pray for them, and they could be healed.

My friend Mary Pat came. She gave me a glass jar filled with cranberries, twigs of pine, white baby's breath, and a single red rose. The jar was simple yet beautiful, like friendship, like God's Invitation.

Mary Pat sat next to me as I cried during the music because it reminded me of my mother. She listened as the pastor's wife, with her sandy blonde hair and bundle of enthusiasm, got up to teach. As Sandi read from the Bible, I imagined a Banquet more wonderful than an Elf feast at Lothlorian, high among the trees.

An Invitation can come in many forms. Recently, a radio station sponsored a Freedom Fest rally in a local mountain meadow. Christian rock bands performed on a huge temporary stage, and booths offered bracelets, t-shirts, hamburgers, iced mochas or free Bibles.

As you know, I've always been a reporter at heart. A few months ago I got a part-time job working for the local newspaper, doing feature articles (with photos) about mountain churches, personalities, and events. It means less time with my books (one reason why this one is taking over three years to write) but a little money and an opportunity to get involved in my community. That's a responsibility and a privilege, as the written word has power to boost business and bring people to events.

My editor said I could cover the Freedom Expo, so I carted my camera and tape recorder around, interviewing friendly members of "Sackcloth Fashion" (a Christian hip-hop band), getting autographs on posters, and taking lots of pictures. Toward evening, when the long shadows from the surrounding pine trees fell on the meadow, a speaker offered an Invitation to the people who sat on blankets on the grass.

And I thought, It must have been like this for Jesus—people following him to meadows, coming for food or entertainment or a message of hope, sitting on the grass with their families and friends, listening.

And I felt God's Spirit sweep down like the wind through pine branches and move among the people. Nearly 50 answered the Invitation and came forward to make a decision for Christ. Whole families, with mom carrying a baby and children at her feet, answered the Invitation. The group gathered near the stage and prayed with Counselors. A little blonde boy of 10, whose parents had just separated, cried his heart out, searching for hope in a hopeless world.

Tears came to my eyes, too, and I felt like I was witnessing a Billy Graham Crusade—on a smaller scale.

Steven Curtis Chapman wrote this song:

"This is your Invitation
Come just the way you are
Come find what your soul has been longing for
Come find your peace
Come find the feast
Come in, this is your Invitation."

How many times must God call before we answer? He has invited us to the greatest Feast of all Time.

To illustrate this, I will tell you about Kristen's wedding to Jeremy, the tall, curly-haired, quiet Christian carpenter she met on her missions trip to Mexico.

We drive down to San Diego for the wedding, taking Jessica and Jonathan, a miniature tuxedo, 2 fancy dresses, a bunch of luggage, a bird cage, and Penny the parrot. We stay at the best-deal hotel we could find through www.hotels.com—a rowdy place on Hotel Circle in Mission Valley.

On Thursday evening, as soon as we get there, I meet Kristen in the lobby. We go out to our last, before-she-gets-married, mother/daughter shopping spree and dinner at Nordstrom. As we sit at the table drinking iced tea and eating large Rice Krispie bars (like old times), I try to give her some practical advice.

"We want to have 3 or 4 children," she says enthusiastically. Her blue eyes are full of innocence and dreams, and her blonde hair hangs over her slender shoulders, exposing one shell-like ear. I can't help but remember when she and I went canoeing on Canim Lake in Canada the year she graduated from high school, not so long ago, and the sunlight shone down on her hair, turning it to gold like a poem about "The Lady of Shallot." And I think,

You've got a lot of pain ahead of you...

Instead I say, "See that woman over there? She's about your age. She's holding a baby. She has been holding that baby, without a break, for the last hour and a half while her friend relaxes and sips on her iced mocha."

Kristen follows my gaze and thinks for a moment.

"Well, maybe we'll wait a couple of years."

And she drops me back at the hotel because she and Jeremy have to meet bridesmaids from Washington where Kristen lived during the time I was going through chemo. And the next morning Jessica and I drive to Costco to get fruit and danishes for the Bridal Shower hosted by Kristen's Maid of Honor, her best friend Beth (whose parents Steve and Karen were our pastors down in the valley while I was going through chemo). And Beth tells the story about how she and Kristen met, one wearing white and the other black, in the famous photo I took when they were fifteen. And Jeremy's mother, a nice lady named Carla who likes to ballroom dance and go on cruises, sits there looking composed while I feel like shouting,

"I'm too young to be a mother-in-law! I'm not ready for this. I have an eight-year-old!"

But instead I behave myself and win the Bridal Shower Game Prize of a coffee-scented candle with little coffee beans stuck all around it in the wax.

And then comes the Rehearsal where I get the name "Mother of the Bride" and walk with Edd to the front of the church. And then the Rehearsal Dinner after, at Jeremy's favorite Chinese restaurant. His mother Carla put bright-colored Beta fish in glass bowls on each table, because Kristen gave a Beta to Jeremy before they started dating, and the poor fish died...

And then the sleepless night and the getting up early and rushing to the church to get dressed. And Edd telling me to calm down and taking Jonathan to the men's dressing area to get his little black tux with a bow tie on so that he resembles a Junior James Bond (I offered to dress Jonathan in his Frodo costume—for what better Ring Bearer could there be—but Kristen refused).

When I walk into the woman's dressing room, I barely recognize Kristen who is getting her makeup done by a friend.

"Mom, you were supposed to be here at 10:00, prompt, already dressed," she tells me.

"I didn't want to wrinkle my dress in the car," I defend. "And it's only seven after. Do you know how long it took me to find a plain royal blue dress in a style I could actually wear to the Renaissance Faire?" I ask.

Kristen shrugs and reaches for her Starbucks coffee. The Makeup Lady finishes up, and I take Kristen's place at the makeup table.

"I don't have time for makeup at home," I explain. "Could you just put a dab here and there?"

"Sure," she says as she gently applies pink eyeshadow.

I watch as bridesmaid Crystal styles Jessie's hair. Jess is a Junior Bridesmaid in a lilac dress (why are most bridesmaid's dresses pastel?). Crystal gives the ten-year-old a lesson in beauty.

"Is that tight enough?" Crystal asks as Jessica clutches the massive hair clip on the back of her head.

"It hurts," Jessie whines.

"Good. Beauty is pain," Crystal replies as she moves on to the next victim—me.

Beth is trying to find a necklace out of the mass of jewelry that Jessica, the third bridesmaid, brought down with her from Washington.

"Do you think this heart looks good?" she asks the room in general. She looks lovely, her strawberry blonde hair curling around her fair face. I feel sad that she has had health problems and tires easily.

"It looks great," I reply as I pull the royal blue dress on.

Jessica and Beth hot-iron Kristen's hair into spiral curls.

"You've got 23 minutes," I tell the bride.

She claps her hands, jumps up and down, and says, "YES!"

Then everyone helps her climb into her dress. It's beautiful, the kind I never had—with crystals and pearls sewn into it, a scoop neck, 3/4 sleeves, lace trimmings, a veil, and a long train.

A man comes into the room with a big black video camera (one of Kristen's uncles on her father's side), shuts the door, and asks if it's OK to be there.

"A man!" I scream, half joking. "Get him out of here."

He stays anyway, to get video of me, with my numb fingers and everyone staring, as I fasten the top 3 buttons on Kristen's wedding gown.

And suddenly I see her at the age of two, with blonde hair in pigtails that bob up and down, and I'm buttoning her pink rosebud sundress before taking her on a walk in our apartment garden to look at the "puty" flowers which she later learned to paint with water colors.

Oh God, I can't cry. I've got to get through this. I'm not ready...

And suddenly it's eleven o'clock, and somehow all the women are ready, and we're lining up outside the church aisle doors, and there's a crowd of people sitting in there on pews waiting for us.

"It's OK," Edd says at my side. I look into his calm, blue-green eyes beneath their massive brows.

Jessica, holds her large bouquet tightly. She's taking her role seriously, about to slowly step down that aisle. Jonathan flirts with the bridesmaids and runs around like a typical eight-year-old.

The music starts, and Ryan, whom I barely recognize in his tuxedo, walks toward me. He adjusts his collar and squirms a little. He leads his stepmother Louise and then comes back to get me. I place my hand on his outstretched arm. He's tall, tanned, his beautiful brown curls cut short because he never liked them and his blue eyes shy. He smiles at me and says, "Relax, Mom."

"You too," I reply.

"Walk slowly," Edd says from behind me, and I step down a different path than I have known.

All six parents of the bride (me, Edd, my ex-husband Jeff, his wife Louise, Jeremy's mother Carla, and Jeremy's new stepdad Dennis) turn to watch the flower girl spread rose petals all around her (she can't figure out how to do it without them falling on her blonde curls). Then Jonathan, smiling like a hobbit, follows, carrying the white lace pillow Beth sewed for him. Then comes the Junior groomsman, a boy Jessica's age. Jess holds onto his arm and steps solemnly, knowing the importance of her role, knowing that after this her big sister will never be the same.

Then the groomsmen and the bridesmaids and the maid of honor. Then a pause, a flourish of music, and Kristen stands there, a vision of white next to her father Jeff.

I burst into tears, and so does Edd.

Kristen smiles ear to ear, her veil draping her back but not covering her face.

"Who gives this woman to be married?" the pastor asks.

"I do," Jeff replies.

He escorts Kristen to her waiting groom and then sits on the other side of Louise, on the same front pew as Edd and I.

The ceremony goes quickly. The Junior Groomsman, who led Jessie down the aisle, forgets to relax his knees and faints. His mother and sisters rush up to him as the Best Man carries him offstage. The ceremony continues, the sound of a siren in the background since someone called 911. Jeremy repeats vows in a soft voice, and Kristen sounds exuberant. They both say "I do." Then they move under a flowered-covered gazebo at the back of the stage and light candles. Two candles become one flame on a wide silver candlestick.

The pastor turns the couple toward the audience and says, "May I introduce Jeremy and Kristen. You may kiss the bride."

Kristen claps her hands again, jumps a little, and slaps her lips onto Jeremy as if to draw his breath away.

My tears have slowed. The photographer got sick and had to leave, so I fill in a little until his assistant takes charge. I take pictures of Jonathan with his big brother Ryan, Jonathan with Jeremy, and Jessica with her sister the bride.

Then the groom and bride leave for the reception, and we all pack up our stuff to follow. I notice that Jeff has been crying, and I walk up to him and ask if he is alright.

"Yes," he says, but I watch him for a moment, his profile against the church window. He is still tall but a little chubbier, with gray along the sides of his head and wrinkles around his pale blue eyes. He wears a sadness in those eyes—for those years gone, for his little girl given to another. And I think,

I'm so sorry I hurt you. Divorce is a terrible thing. It always brings pain.

True, the divorce wasn't all my fault. Jeff fits much better with Louise than crazy me, and I'm much more like Edd. Kristen has more family than she would have—and lots more presents. But does that take away the pain?

At the reception, which Jeff and Louise host, we see San Diego bay through big plate windows, and sailboats gliding by. The tables are filled with flowers, white china, silver settings, and crystal goblets. Edd, the kids, and I are at Table Three. The wedding party sits on a long row up front. After relaxing for awhile and eating prime rib, Beth says a toast,

"I'm glad that Jeremy and Kristen met while serving the Lord, building houses in Mexico." She pauses and glances at Ryan, whom she has liked for years. He smiles back. "I never thought construction could be so romantic. I should try it sometime."

Jeff says a naval officer toast, appropriate and funny. Edd says that he remembers meeting Kristen when she was Jessica's age, and how proud he is of her and Jeremy serving the Lord.

Ryan gets up, sweaty in his black tux jacket, and says between tears,

"When we were children, she was my older sister, and I always followed her around. Now I realize that we are no longer children, and I can't follow her anymore..."

He can't finish his toast for the tears, and sits down. Edd comes to the rescue with a joke.

I look at my oldest son who was hurt most by my divorce and think,

You can still follow her, Ryan.

And then I take a mic, staring out at people dressed in their best clothes, sparkling, formal, quiet—all eyes on me.

"I'm a writer, and I usually have lots to say," I mumble, tears at the back of my eyes. "I just want to thank Jeremy and Kristen for giving us a symbol of Christ's love for the church—and how our banquet will be in Heaven someday."

I hold up my glass of sparkling apple cider as an Invitation.

The Christian DJ opens the dance floor. Edd leads me out for a slow dance, clutching my small hand in his large one and guiding my feet across the parquet floor. He holds me closer, and the music swirls around us.

"I love you," he whispers in my ear as his beard tickles my cheek. I fit well in the circle of his arms.

Kristen and Jeremy dance to our right, Ryan and Beth dance to our left, Jessica dances with the Junior Groomsman who fainted but has recovered, and little Jonathan dances with two tall bridesmaids at once.

The music takes a faster beat, and we spin and loop and kick up our heels. Kristen has abandoned her veil, attached the long train to the back of her wedding dress, and exchanged her delicate white sandals for tennis shoes so that she can dance with all her heart—with her groom, her family, and the wedding guests. I hope to be as excited as Kristen the Bride when I arrive at the Banquet to Come:

"He brought me to the banqueting house,
 and his banner over me was love." (Song of Solomon 2:4)

"Blessed are those who are called
to the marriage supper of the Lamb!" (Revelation 19:9)

"And the Spirit and the bride say, 'Come!'
And let him who hears say, 'Come!'
And let him who thirsts come.
Whoever desires, let him take
the water of life freely." (Revelation 22:17)

Postscripts

Land of the Silver Fern

Things don't always turn out as you imagine.

Doris Bowers, whom I had pretty much given up on, rallied over the summer. Her cancer went into remission, and she started hiking and teaching her nature classes again.

My friend Cherie (who had given birth to a stillborn son) moved off the mountain, along with her husband, new baby, and four other kids. Of all places, they moved to the hot desert of Arizona.

Jessica and Jonathan gave up figure skating.

And we flew off to New Zealand.

⁂

Ever since we saw Peter Jackson's first <u>Lord of the Rings</u> movie, we had wanted to see the land where it was filmed—the islands farther south than Australia, where Penguins migrate from their Antarctic home, glacial mountains keep their snow, and jungles stay green year-round. Then we met Liz and her family at Carlsbad, who invited us to stay with them in Wellington. So we called up our timeshare company and amazingly got two weeks at Lake Taupo.

The scorching California summer heat, drought, and bark

beetles had caused the pine trees on our mountain to die and become towers of brown kindling. The mountains reached 100 degrees, and the valley smog levels rose. Fire warnings and evacuation plans filled the newspaper where I had got a part-time job. The governor declared our mountains a disaster zone and sought state and federal aid to cut down the dead trees.

It was winter in New Zealand. There was plenty of rain, lakes, rivers, and green trees. The islands beckoned to us. I never thought I would be glad to leave my beloved mountains. On August 1st, friends from Calvary Chapel drove us to the airport.

Edd, Jessica, Jonathan, and I endured a 13-hour flight which took us 10,500 kilometers and crossed the Equator and International Date Line. We arrived at Auckland in the middle of the night, stunned, disoriented, exhausted, but excited over the new land that lay before us, ready for exploration.

We had come to Middle-earth, On the Trail of the Ring, but we found much more than we expected.

Immediately we realized we had too much luggage as we waited in the long Customs line where a beagle dog sniffed suitcases for food or honey. A guard checked the bottoms of my hiking boots to make sure I wasn't bringing in biological items like grass, twigs, or dirt. A clerk stamped our blue American passports, and we were free to explore the airport and haggle with the rental car attendant.

The first moment we stepped through the glass doors towards a lawn by the parking lot, a bird's song filled the night air. The song, one I had never heard before, lilted up and down and clearly called, "Tui, Tui!" as a welcome to us. I could not see the bird in the branches of the strange, bushy tree. Edd called me forward as I paused to stare up at dark leaves. A few steps later I paused again to look up at the clear night sky full of unfamiliar stars. The Southern Cross hovered at the Zenith like God's blessing on the land.

That is when I first began to lose my heart...

Jessica and Jonathan, behind me, asked what the stars meant. I told them they formed a cross and added, "You can see them only from beneath the Equator."

We smelled salt air from the nearby sea. Even though we were near a large city, this was probably the freshest air we had ever breathed.

We found our small, expensive rental car and piled our luggage in. After we all got our seatbelts on, Edd announced, "I don't know how to turn the headlights on." I went to ask a taxi driver for help, and the Tui bird sang again.

Edd remembered how to drive on the left side of the road and through Roundabouts, as he had done on our visit to England before the children were born. I tried to figure out the map, and we got to the nearby motel at 1:00 in the morning New Zealand time (6:00 in the morning California time, on the previous day). The modest motel (which I found through www.hotels.com) had an office, a lawn, some trees, and glass all along the front of our room, Polynesian-style.

Edd hauled in the necessary luggage, and we fell asleep only to awaken to a very bright sun—too late for visiting Calvary Chapel of Auckland.

The room had a small kitchen with a mini fridge and a little carton of milk for the teabags and coffee spread out for us. We used the electric tea kettle to make our hot drinks and sat around a small round table, munching on health bars I had carried in my laptop case (yes, I had declared them at Customs).

Nothing ever tasted as good as that tea.

Then we got to take a shower. The knobs were backwards, and even the water swirled in the opposite direction down the drain. But the warm water felt wonderful after the cramped, stale, sweaty airplane. After we were all dressed and packed again, I got out our map. We stared at it and thought, Where do we go first?

The North and South Islands, filled with unfamiliar names (both Maori and English), spread out before us in blue and green and black.

"Let's go straight to Taupo," Edd decided. "It's only about four hours South, and our timeshare room is waiting for us."

We all agreed, packed up, and turned in the expensive rental car for a cheaper one through a local company.

"No worries," the cheerful attendant told us as she gave us more maps and helped us load our luggage. "This will do you fine."

We headed for Highway One, South toward Hamilton, deciding not to go north into Auckland city. Only a few minutes from the airport the landscaped changed from suburban houses and shopping centers to emerald green hills and farmland. At every new vista of sweeping pastures I wanted to yell, "Stop here! We're in The Shire! Let me unpack Jonathan's Frodo costume, his ring, and his plastic sword! Let me dress him up and take his photo in front of those hills!"

But I knew there would be a month of opportunities, so I stayed silent, the map on my knees as Edd drove along the Waikato River to a little town called Huntly where we stopped for shopping and lunch.

We took our first photo there, on the grassy banks of the wide river, near willow trees, black swans, yellow flowers, and a hawk. We ate our first minced meat pies with chips and pots of strong tea. We shopped for postcards of mountains, lakes, jungles, volcanoes, and seashores. We bought blue-green paua shells; a stuffed Kiwi bird; and black t-shirts embroidered with the Silver Fern. We touched smooth Maori artwork—bone or jade carved into oval pendants.

Everyone we met was polite, with a lilting accent and cheerful tone. They seemed interested in where we were from and what stories we could tell them. I told complete strangers I was a cancer survivor, gave them my business card, and asked them to check out my website. I even gave away copies of my books (that had taken up one whole suitcase, much to Edd's annoyance).

After lunch, we turned west and drove through higher hills covered with thick evergreen forests. Deep shade lurked under thick boughs, beckoning us to stop and explore their paths.

"Mommie, there are huge ferns under those trees," Jessica observed, pointing. "I want to get out and touch them."

I agreed with her, glimpsing green fronds caught by the afternoon sun as we sped past. Our two-lane highway was well paved but had no center divider or shoulder rails, so we couldn't drive past 100 kilometers per hour.

The hills became more rugged —cliffs topped by jagged rocks which could have been the setting for Weathertop in <u>The Fellowship of the Ring</u>. We passed lakes and rivers, their water glistening in sunlight —clear, unpolluted, flowing over mossy stones.

"When will we be there?" Jonathan asked from his little spot in the back seat where suitcases and winter coats surrounded him.

"Soon," Edd replied, his face stuck ahead on the road as the yellow divider lines swept past.

We had packed for a cold, snowy winter and wore our sheepskin boots, wool traveling pants, and hooded jackets. But so far the air felt refreshingly cool, and we rolled the car windows down to let it bathe our faces. We saw no snow as we traveled south toward Lake Taupo.

We passed a Maori village surrounded by steaming hot springs and bubbling pools, where I wanted to stop and explore, but Edd urged us onward, wanting to get to Taupo before dark. We passed geothermal plants with steam rising in great plumes out of the volcanic earth. Then we came to a hilltop that overlooked Lake Taupo. We got out and marveled at the size of the lake—at least 50 miles long. At the far end rose the volcanic mountains of Tongariro National Park, covered with snow and clouds.

"Ooooh!" I exclaimed, almost jumping in excitement as I lifted my arms to stretch.

Edd easily found the Taupo Ika Nui, our timeshare resort. Right across from the lake, it had a garden filled with native New Zealand plants. After we checked in at the office, we found a little sign the gardener had painted:

"If you're lonesome for your own garden, please pick the odd weed."

I never was good with gardens. My garden is a California

National Forest. But I thought, maybe I could grow something in a place like this.

We unloaded the whole car and filled the little one-bedroom condo with our many suitcases and winter coats.

"I knew I shouldn't have brought this guitar," Edd grumbled as he leaned it against a wall. But later he took it out and serenaded us all to sleep as the Southern Cross shone in the pure dark sky above.

The next two weeks, with Taupo as our base, we explored as much of the North Island as our energy and time allowed.

We watched boats take tourists out for "a spot of trout fishing" on the lake (this being the trout capital of the world). We looked through brochures, watched the New Zealand news, and ate good chocolate. We shopped in town, exploring stores full of treasures like native wood carved into fish shapes by Maori craftsmen, who add pieces of bluegreen paua (abalone shell) to represent bright eyes. We went to a bakery where they cut the loaf you order and bought fresh vegetables at a store called Pumpkin Planet, across from the park which had a huge public bathroom called The Super Loo, that had lockers, showers, and a children's room.

We chatted with shop owners who had been Orcs in The Lord of the Rings films. We made friends with the managers of the Taupo Ika Nui (who kept giving us toilet paper and coffee packets). We met a family in a condo near ours, whose children Jonathan played with in the courtyard. Tim had been a Rider of Rohan, and he liked to sit on his balcony and watch Lake Taupo through binoculars. His wife Terri invited me up on the balcony for tea, and I gave her a copy of my chemo book.

"We're from Hastings, near Napier," Tim told me. "I like to play Rugby."

"And I'm a full-time mum," Terri added, picking up my book to glance at the cover.

We found a little cafe with no name, where you could pick your minced meat pie or shepherd's pie or toasted sandwiches and eat them (with cafe latte or pots of tea) while sitting in green canvas chairs at round tables on the sidewalk. We chatted with Jodie the Maori waitress from Auckland who had just moved to Taupo.

"I am so glad to get out of the city," she confided. "I love this little town in the country. Have you seen The Hidden Valley?"

"Not yet," Edd replied.

"No worries," she said with a smile. "I'll give you a map. There's a lovely fern grotto there, and a lake by some hot springs. The ferryman takes you across."

That sounded interesting, so we spent an afternoon looking for The Hidden Valley, finding it along an old logging road, and relaxing on the dock by the large clear lake surrounded by hills. Jessica and Jonathan oohed and aaahed over the huge rainbow trout that swam in clear water right up to the dock. Then Jessica showed us the black swans in the shallows by willow trees, their black feathers arched up along their backs and their red beaks parting to sing their low, sad song.

Another day, we hiked along the steaming mineral springs that flow into the Waikato River. I snapped a photo of a tree with steam drifting up through its branches while sunlight shone down, lighting each leaf, clearly etching it against the white mist. We walked further, pausing to dip our feet into the hot water that bubbles down a waterfall into a pool where hikers bathe. We walked through thermal Craters of the Moon where active volcanic steam rushes out of the earth in pillars of sulfur. Nothing grows at the hottest parts of those craters, which plunge many feet into the earth. The mud along the bottom boils noisily, reminding you to stay upon the path. Along the edges of the craters, hardy moss and ferns somehow thrive in the acidic soil.

This would be a geologist's or a botanist's dreamland.

Edd humored me as I finally got to dress Jonathan up in his green Frodo cape with its gold oakleaf clasp. I snapped his photo in front of a farmer's hilly field which we found on our way to the west coast. The setting transformed Jonathan from an eight-year-old American boy into Little Frodo. Sunlight shone down upon him, highlighting his little hand that held a gold-hilt sword; his ring; his beautiful face with blue eyes and curly hair—the face that looked as serious as a hobbit bound to carry the Ring of Doom.

"Maybe you're overdoing this a bit," Edd suggested. "We don't want the child to have nightmares."

I thought about his observation and took the ring off the chain Jonathan wore around his neck. I replaced it with a pewter shield that had a cross on one side and a verse on the other: "Be strong and of good courage; do not be afraid, nor be dismayed, for the LORD your God is with you wherever you go."

"That's better," I admitted as I unhooked the green cape and put Jonathan's red jacket back on.

But I knew I would like that photo I had taken, and I would use my new white Macintosh iBook laptop computer to email it, along with the story of our New Zealand trip, to my editor back in the California mountains. I did that on a rainy night in Taupo, with the help of an Internet Cafe and a very patient Kiwi computer whiz.

One day, Jessica and I left Edd and Jonathan in the condo where they were content to listen to music CDs and play the guitar. We went horseback riding through an ancient forest filled with evergreens, big-leaved plants, and ferns (New Zealand has so many different ferns that they require a separate nature book). The winter air felt chilly, it rained a little, and there weren't many flowers in bloom. But everything looked green and alive—like Middle-earth should be. Jessica felt like Arwin the Elf Princess while she galloped through a clearing, the fresh air in her face as she urged her horse faster.

A couple of hours after that, Jess and I went kayaking on the Waikato River. Our guide, The River Man, knew the Waikato well and told us stories of how you can paddle all the way to the sea. He avoided Huka Falls, telling us that a kayaker would not survive its rocky rapids. He showed us the tree swing you could climb to from the bank and launch over the river, to let go and plunge your body into the refreshing current. He showed us the bungie jumpers on cliffs high above, elastic ropes tied to their ankles as they dove down to where even their heads went underwater and people in boats had to haul them out. He let us beach the boats and soak in the hot spring waterfalls next to a footpath. When we climbed back into the kayaks, I felt like Galadriel in a graceful Elvish boat as I paddled with the current, treeboughs overhanging both banks of the river and the water making graceful elvish swirls around me.

One day, Edd decided to check out the East Coast. We drove through forest lands along Highway 5 to Napier, a coastal city that was destroyed by an earthquake in the 1930s and rebuilt Art Deco style. We walked on a black-pebbled beach while fierce green breakers crashed behind us. We drove by the Sea Aquarium then headed back toward Hawke's Bay which is bordered by hilly farmland and vineyards. I snapped a photo of the eastern farmland panorama with a river gorge in the background. Jessica and Jonathan were glad to get out of the car to wander in a farmer's high pasture, the green turf so thick they could bounce on it.

"I want to go for a walk," Jess pleaded.

"Another time," Edd said.

And I remembered England, when I took Kristen and Ryan to North Yorkshire. They were about the same ages as Jessica and Jonathan—and we tramped across the moors all day.

We climbed back into the car, ate cookies, chocolate, and cheese—and continued driving up Highway 5. I got the brilliant idea to return on Route 38 westward, not realizing that the dirt road was remote, narrow, and wet. It rose high above Lake Waikaremoana where there were no guardrails to keep one from plummeting down steep cliffs. It wound through a jungle, by flooding rivers, and past an occasional cow that strayed into the road. Darkness fell before we reached the paved highway, and Edd swore he would not take another shortcut even though I used my green laser light to mark the way ahead.

⁂

Edd broke his rule a few days later when we went to the West Coast. At least the road was paved. It wound past woods where the tall, native trees called Rimu rose above the others, their peeling silvery trunks glistening in the sun. Herds of wooly sheep dotted hilly green farmland (there are seven sheep for every person in New Zealand). We found another lake with cliffs towering above it, a little town called Bennydale, and the famous limestone caves of Waitomo where we examined stalactites and stalagmites in one cave and glowworms above an underground river in another. The glowworms lit up the dark rock ceiling with tiny blue lights in their tails, attracting prey to their dangling "feeder lines." Even Edd was impressed as our boat glided silently beneath the starry sight.

A high, narrow road led through more sheepland to the little village of Marokopa on the wild Western Coast. Here the tempestuous Tasman Sea separates New Zealand from Australia. We walked on magnetic black sand, along the banks of a river that flowed into breaking ocean waves. Lava rocks and limestone cliffs rose as shoreline behind us, and the sun set in a blaze of pink and orange over a dark-blue sea.

When we drove back after dark, the Silver Fern lined the high-banked road. Its underside caught the car's headlamps in a band of silver light as if to guide us. The Maori people bend the dark green fern so that its silver underside glows in the moonlight, and the fernpoints mark a path through the forest.

As we headed back to Taupo through silent hills, the moon shone full above us. Mars, at its closest point to earth, glowed red beneath the moon. I thought about J.R.R. Tolkien, the English professor of ancient languages who never journeyed to the South Pacific. He imagined an elvish forest with trees lit up by silver lights and called it Lothlorian.

You can find it in New Zealand.

※

A few days later, we journeyed south of Taupo to Tongariro National Park and its snowy volcanic mountains that we had seen from the other side of the lake.

We drove past evergreen forests, rivers, and a strange, orange-brown grassland cut through with jagged black volcanic rocks—a fitting scene for Mordor.

We drove to to highest peak, Mount Ruapehu. An active volcano, it rises 8000 feet above Lake Taupo and is joined by the two other mountains of Tongariro National Park. We could see steam rising from their slopes. Hot springs and eerie milk-blue lakes hide in their heights.

We passed The Grand Chalet, an old-style hotel surrounded by grassland, streams, and hiking trails. A few kilometers up another road brought us to the Whakapapa Ski Fields.

We arrived on a sunny day and found our first snow of New Zealand. The children looked like Polar bears in their matching silver parkas and snow boots as they stomped in drifts and threw snowballs. We breathed in the brisk, cold air and took more photos. Edd bought lift tickets, and we rode to the top, wondering how the people below us could navigate among sharp rocks and cliffs.

We changed from the Centennial to the Waterfall Express which took us close to the Summit, where skiers catch the T-bar to the highest runs. We explored the cafe and shop, then watched the skiers and snowboarders through plate-glass windows as we sipped hot tea. One plucky girl in pink, about 10 years old, kept going down the most difficult run.

"If you can ski Ruapehu, you can ski any mountain in the world," a Kiwi grandma at the next table told us. "I learned to ski at 58."

We began to understand why New Zealand is known for its extreme sports.

As we rode down the lift, the mountains and valley spread

out below us in a panorama dotted by clouds. Jonathan, sitting next to me, gripped the metal safety bar with both hands and said, "I'm not afraid anymore. I want to learn to ski."

Jessica, who sat in the front chair with Edd, screamed with joy and terror as we skimmed above black crags, level with a harrier hawk and the snowy crater top.

※

After two weeks in Taupo, we drove down to visit my friend Liz in Wellington. The day started out cool and rainy, and because of an accident on Highway 1, we had to loop around Tongariro National Park where we glimpsed Mount Ruapehu from all angles. We drove through farmland, river gorges, coastal towns, and old villages before arriving just before dark. When we pulled up to Liz's nice suburban home in the hills north of Wellington, we were greeted by her shy smile as she emerged from her doorway.

Liz reminded me so much of myself: shoulder-length blonde hair, blue eyes, and a habit of wearing silver pendants on green sweaters, over black pants and sheepskin boots. Liz was an English major in college, read my favorite books, and even used the same face soap. I joked that she was my New Zealand twin (more reserved, of course).

Her daughters Johanna and Olivia were as cute as ever with their brown shy eyes and bobbed brunette hair. Andrew was away on a business trip to Washington D.C. for the first day, so Liz helped us get settled in her spare room. We had a little time before dark to admire her garden that was already blooming with yellow flowers from the native Kowhai tree.

Unlike me, Liz liked to cook. I was impressed by her kitchen and New Zealand ingenuity—that Americans could learn from. Liz had an oven with a setting for convection, where fans made the heat more efficient so that meals cooked quicker. Her double dishwasher could be set for two separate loads at different times (and, of course, used less water and electricity than American dishwashers). The cheese cutter was long and white, with two sides like a double-edged sword. The electric plastic teakettle made water boil faster than a metal one heated on a stovetop. I watched, fascinated, as Liz cooked.

She served dinner in her formal dining room complete with place settings that had different photos of New Zealand on them. She made a typical Kiwi meal: roast lamb on a platter with yams, potatoes, and carrots; peas; salad; and Pavlova for desert (Pavlova is baked meringue topped with whipped cream and kiwi fruit). After dinner we chatted and watched the All Blacks rugby team beat Australia. The big, rough players wore black shorts and shirts—with the silver fern emblazoned on their hearts.

The next morning we had a typical New Zealand breakfast of cereal and fruit, then took the soggy green footpath to Liz's neighborhood Anglican church. We immediately felt at home with the calvary-chapel-style music (guitars and praise songs). The friendly people greeted us curiously (not seeing many Americans in their church service) and passed around a book for us to write prayer requests in.

"We could tell you were Americans before you said a thing," one woman told me. "Because of your foot gear."

I looked down at our feet and chuckled because we were all wearing winter boots, and they were wearing dress shoes or sandals.

We took our seats, and Pastor Danny, who was half Maori, spoke with the enthusiasm of a man dedicated to the Lord and to his community.

"Only 10 percent of New Zealanders go to church," he said. "What an opportunity to reach out to the other 90 percent!"

After his sermon, he and the altar boys shared Communion with us, stopping before each of us to say with meaning,

"The blood of Christ which was shed for you."

After the service Liz went to her prayer group while the children played outside. Edd and I lingered to speak with Pastor Danny and his wife Linda. Danny told us how he gave up a lucrative engineering career to become a minister. Edd shared how he led worship at our Calvary Chapel back home.

"We really love New Zealand," I said as I handed Pastor Danny my card.

Andrew, a tall, quiet man with brown hair and glasses, had arrived home from his long flight but was too tired to accompany us on a tour of Wellington (he works for a navigation software company that is way ahead of America). So, after lunch, the rest of us piled into Liz's van and visited the seaside area where Peter Jackson has a home near The Chocolate Fish Cafe. We stopped at the overcrowded landmark for coffee and little chocolate fish filled with green marshmallow. Then we walked down the street to Jackson's house, feeling a little stupid, and peered over the brick wall. Good thing nobody was home. We saw kids' bicycles and other toys laying in the yard, and a lonely dog brought a stick for us to play with.

Liz showed us the elementary school that Peter Jackson's kids attend and the seaside bluff which was the setting for the town of Bree. One rainy night, the hobbits fled the ringwraiths there and found refuge in The Prancing Pony Inn, where they first met the hooded Aragorn. Who would have thought that the dark, walled town was so close to the sea!

We got out near Bree and walked by the beach while the four children romped on a playground. Then Liz drove us up foresty Mount Victoria, a large park in the middle of Wellington, where some of the first film scenes were shot. We climbed to the top and looked all around at seaports, skyscrapers, bays, the airport, and seaside villages. The children climbed an old cannon for a photo, and Liz drove us down into the city which was full of one-way streets, tall buildings, and interesting shops. We saw the official Lord of the Rings bookstore (where they sell action figures) and Te Papa, the National Museum, where you can buy a replica of the leaf pin the Lothlorian elves gave to the Fellowship of Nine.

Liz ended our excursion with a ride of the cable car which ended on a hill topped with gardens.

"You'd make a good tour guide," I told her as we drove back to her house after dark.

She only smiled at me, and I wondered what she thought of

brash Californians.

Liz and Andrew spent the evening looking at digital photos on my laptop computer while the children played "Zoo Tycoon" software on the corner desktop. Andrew downloaded some of my digital photos, then he and Edd watched the video of the previous night's All Blacks game. Andrew explained the meaning of the "huka" Maori wardance the team performs before each game (complete with grunts, yells, and mean faces). Somehow Andrew (who is an electrical engineer) made time to help Johanna and Jonathan build a Morris Code telegraph machine with an electrical kit. Liz served tea again, and we adults chatted until bedtime while the children took care of their virtual zoo.

"Did you know that in New Zealand many of the public schools still allow prayer and Bible classes?" Liz asked.

"That's true especially on the South Island," Andrew added. "It depends upon the district and who's in charge."

Edd and I found this information amazing. Maybe I wouldn't Homeschool if we lived in New Zealand.

We said goodnight to a tired Liz and Andrew and took the kids upstairs to bed.

Monday morning Liz had a full schedule with her children and household duties, and Andrew had to go to work for a meeting. We helped ourselves to breakfast, then barely saw Liz enough to thank her before heading to catch the Blue Bridge ship to The South Island.

I didn't feel ready to leave, because we had no idea where we would be staying, and we would be driving from place to place like gypsies. But the restful 3 1/2 hours on an ocean liner (with a cafe, observation room, open decks, and our own private stateroom complete with beds and sink) gave us a chance to nap before discovering the most beautiful parts of New Zealand.

How do I begin describing the South Island? The locals say it is more beautiful the further south you go. But the top of the island was breathtaking, with long fingers of forested land cut by water channels. When we docked at Picton, the man who helped unload our luggage remarked, "Where is the kitchen sink?" and we wished again we had brought half the stuff.

We drove south along the east coast as evening fell, along wave-beaten stretches of rocky beach with snowy mountains above them. We ended our drive in Kaikoura, where the rental car lady had recommended a clean new cottage near the beach. An American, Suzi from Oregon, ran the cottage with her Kiwi husband. She showed us the beautiful house with two bedrooms, a large kitchen, living room, dining room, and shiny wood floors. Exhausted from the sea voyage and four-hour drive, we did not hesitate to say we would stay for three nights (for which she gave us a discount).

The next morning, sunlight illumined the long stretch of curving beach and the white mountains behind it. The children hunted for smooth rocks and seashells, and we went into town to discover the essentials: the fish 'n chips shop, the pharmacy, the market, the bakery, and the bank. We would have plenty of time to explore the tourist gift and jewelry shops later. The village was one long strip next to the beach and reminded us of some old California beachtowns.

While we were in Kaikoura, Jessica wanted me to take her horseback riding again. This time it would be a two-hour trek along a river. I agreed, and we left Jonathan safely with Edd while we drove toward the green hills that backed up to the snowy mountains.

Our guide, Pete, was dressed like an American cowboy—complete with white felt hat, boots, a handlebar mustache, and a sheathed knife clipped to a leather belt with a large silver buckle. Pete, who was probably in his late 50s but as fit as a much younger man, greeted us with a broad Kiwi drawl and the first of many funny stories. He gave us horses to ride (not ponies)—very tall horses that used to race, with English hunter-style saddles.

I could barely pull myself into the saddle of my horse, and then I had to hold onto it because the horse kept wanting to canter at a very fast pace, though Pete (enjoying my plight) would yell back at me:

"Keep your reins up! Hands off the saddle! Where did you learn how to ride? You had better give up working with computers all day; they'll kill you."

We crossed the shallow, rocky river and rode along a trail bordered by bushes (not many ferns in the South Island). Pete gave us a good lesson on English riding, especially how to hold our thumbs over the reins.

"Two things are important in riding," he lectured. "How you hold the reins and how you keep your balance in the saddle."

I noticed that he had a large Western-style saddle with stirrups much easier to keep one's boots in.

When we pulled the horses up to the river for a photo shot, he asked what the "Crimson Mercy" emblem on my jacket meant. I told him that it was a Christian rock band.

"I didn't know those two words could go together," he replied.

I tried to explain all about Calvary Chapel worship music, and he replied,

"Our national religion is rugby."

I spent the rest of the ride trying not to fall off my horse. Jessie did very well, straight in her saddle like an expert, her long braid hanging down her back.

※

From Kaikoura, we took day trips inland toward those beckoning mountains. We followed a road that went through more rolling green hills (covered with sheep and cows) to the foot of Mount Lyford, where we stopped at a big wooden lodge. The lodge had a high fireplace, and I made Jonathan wear his Frodo costume for a picture in front of its flame (though he got so hot he frowned in the picture). The bartender was sniffling and admitted to us that he had drunk too much Steinlager the night before, and nothing tasted good.

"Besides, I'm getting a cold," he whined.

I stared at the whisky behind him, poured in different-shaped and colored bottles that made them look inviting. One bottle was a bright blue color, like whiskey from another planet. All along another side of the bar were taps for ales and beers, and green and gold beer bottles lined one shelf against a mirror.

How easily we are hooked in...

"Drink some hot tea with lemon and honey," I suggested, pointing to a steel teapot. I wondered why the boss would hire an alcoholic as a bartender. "And stop drinking that other stuff. It will kill you. It killed both my parents."

He stared at me, and I explained to him about Christ's death and resurrection to save us, telling a little of my own story.

"You need to give your life to the Lord. Is there a church around here?" I asked, surprising myself because I am not usually that bold with strangers.

"I think there's one in the next village," he replied with a sniffle.

"Well, here's my card. You could visit my website and read the rest of my story. There are lots of nice photos, too," I suggested, handing him the small invitation.

He stared at the photo on it (Kristen dressed up as Miranda, the future teenager from <u>Like a Tree Planted</u>, her hands entwined in a eucalyptus tree).

"Maybe I will."

As if to offer something in return for the advice, the bartender sold us muffins and tea at half price. When we left, he still looked miserable, haunched over the bar, his eyes and nose red, and his skin pallid.

We drove on down the lonely road and passed that village. The church was an old stone one with a scary-looking English-style graveyard around it (the kind with big headstones covered with lichen and tilting to one side). That church looked like it hadn't been used in awhile, except for funerals. I imagined it filled with Christian rock music, sunlight, and people overflowing onto its old stone steps.

Edd was sick of driving, but I convinced him to go the distance to Hamner Springs, since Liz had recommend it. So we went up a high mountain bridge (where people were bungie-jumping), past a rushing river that offered white water rafting and jet boating, and through a wide valley to an area of natural hot springs where, for a small fee, we could use the various mineral spas or a swimming pool with giant waterslides (which the kids had fun on).

Our swimsuits came in handy after all, but we didn't need to bring that snorkle gear.

⁂

From Kaikoura we drove south down a stormy coast. At one bend in the road I saw a flock of penguins standing together on a small beach that was surrounded by black rocks.

"Look!" I said, but we drove by too fast for anyone else to see them.

We avoided Christchurch (not wanting to stay in a city) and headed to the Inland Canterbury area, landing in a pretty little town called Geraldine. Geraldine was built by the English in the 1800s, to reflect an English village complete with flowering trees and gardens winding by a river. We ate dinner at the old hotel, which had high carved ceilings, chandeliers, dormer windows, and plush red carpet like some places I remember in Yorkshire. We got good deals in the local crafters' shop, buying watercolors of the nearby mountains—including one of Mount Sunday where Edoras, the walled city of Rohan, was built.

We spent the next day driving along Inland Scenic Route 72, next to the Rangitata River Gorge and a snowy mountain range, looking for Mount Sunday. The site of Edoras turned out to be a heap of red rocks at the end of a long gravely road. How Peter Jackson got all his equipment and crew down that road amazed me, since our car barely made it.

Tired of driving on muddy, rutted roads, we ended up in Methven, at the foot of Mount Hutt (a well-known ski area). The town looked deserted though it wasn't very late, and we ended up in a cheerful old yellow pub where we were the only customers. The barmaid, a young skier from Australia, informed us that Mount Hutt was really called Mount Shut because it was closed more than it was open (due to windy conditions, too little, or too much snow). She brought us some hot soup and sandwiches, then went to clean the bar until more customers entered, sat down, and ordered drinks. She brought out a whole tray of glasses and dropped it. All the thick mugs shattered on the stone floor.

Embarrassed, she cleaned up the mess while the people who had ordered the drinks watched her silently. Later, I walked over to the shiny wood bar with its array of unbroken glasses on the wall behind it, and tried to console her by mentioning what a klutz I am and how I try to stay out of kitchens.

"I've been here all winter, working the bar more than skiing," she confided, close to tears. "But maybe things will change, and the mountain will open up."

"No worries," I said, handing her my card with a smile and inviting her to visit my website.

༄

Tired of the relatively high accommodation prices in Geraldine, we drove southwest to Mackenzie District, on a narrow road through sheepland, forests, and mountains. We stopped in a farming town in a wide valley that was surrounded by green hills with higher snowy peaks behind them. The town was one long road of wooden shops and hotels, with a golf course and park at one end and a war memorial on the other. The nearby mountains had ski fields, but we didn't see many skiers.

"Let's check the Tourist Information Bureau for a place to stay," Edd suggested, stopping out front of the brick building. It was a library turned into a pub and part-time Information

Center.

I ran in and asked the barmaid for help, and she directed me to the back wall where brochures were stacked and posters hung by locals who rented out a room or cottage. There on the wall was a sign for "Possum Cottage," on a nearby sheep farm. The rates were reasonable, so I called the name on the poster, and a friendly-sounding woman said that we could rent the cottage for a few days—just give her time to clean it up after the previous occupants.

Late afternoon, we drove down a long dirt road to the very end where green pastures rose into snow-dusted hills. We parked the car and admired the large, modern farmhouse with its skylights and high wood ceilings (made with wood from their own land). A wide porch spread around the house, and near the front door lay muddy coats and boots. To the right, the computer room blazed with light as a girl about Jessica's age sat at a monitor and keyboard. We knocked on the big wooden door, and Sonia, the farmer's wife, met us.

A muscular-looking woman about my age, she had short brown hair streaked with blonde, pronounced cheekbones, green eyes, and a shy smile. She handed us an old-fashioned key (which we really didn't need) and walked with us down the path, past the toolshed and garage, to Possum Cottage. It was the original old farmhouse and had a fence around it, a lawn with bushes and trees, a carport, shed, and a back gate that led to streams and footpaths.

Inside, the cottage had a charming old kitchen filled with mismatched china and odds and ends of food left by travelers. The dining room windows overlooked the eastern fields and had an old formica table and chairs out of the 1950s. The master bedroom had windows all around it and a hardwood floor with a sheepskin to sink one's feet in. There were wooden shelves with various knickknacks like miniature animals and teacups. Two other bedrooms, with several twin-sized beds, could accommodate two large families. The living room had a fireplace and a painted wood mantel adorned by candles; a bookshelf; and comfy warm sofas with big pillows.

Edd quickly started a fire, since it was rainy and cold (and the fireplace also warmed the water heater). I wanted to take a bath in the large old bathtub (most of our New Zealand bathrooms had only showers). We turned the electric heater on in the kids' room (the old-fashioned type like my grandmother used to have—large white tubes once run by steam). The farmer's teenage son brought us a bottle of propane for the portable gas heater. After unpacking and sitting by the fire and drinking hot tea, we felt warm again.

The rain had stopped, and there was still light enough in the sky to see the green pastures that rose behind Possum Cottage, so the kids and I pulled on our snowboots and went for a twilight walk. We carefully shut the gate behind us and walked across an old, slippery bridge above a running stream that had its source in the snowy hills above. We slipped on the muddy path, glad for once that we brought those boots. We climbed higher, toward a lone cabbage tree that stood in the middle of a high field. After examining that tree (which was surrounded by rocks so that the sheep wouldn't eat it), we climbed higher, through taller grass toward a line of evergreens and the top gate that led to the snowy part of the hills, next to a tree-lined ravine cut by the stream.

"We could hike right into the snow," I said, pausing with my hand on the gatelatch.

"But it's getting dark," Jessica replied in a worried voice.

"Let's keep going!" Jonathan urged.

I looked back the way we had come. It seemed steeper going down. All around us was the vast valley, cut by rivers and lakes, lined by pastures and hills. To the north and west the high mountains showed off their deep drifts of snow against the dark sky in which stars had begun to shine.

Jessica had pinned her sapphire light to her belt, so she shined a blue path for us down the hillside. As the three of us bounced down toward Possum Cottage, where light blazed out the windows and Edd waited by the fire, I thought again of England. Kristen and Ryan were Jessica and Jonathan's age when I took them to North Yorkshire where we explored the open moors together.

When we got back to the farm, I stopped and said, "Listen."

We were among a double row of trees that looked like a mix of eucalyptus and firs. They were filled with unseen birds that sang the closing of the day. As we stood still, we were surrounded by a symphony of music—the magpie with her flute-like melody, the Tui bird calling its name, sparrows with their simple notes, and many other birds we did not know.

In the failing light I could see the children's faces glowing, their eyes lit with wonder at the New Zealand countryside, and their mouths curved into smiles of simple joy.

༄

Our days in Possum cottage—in Mackenzie District, in the middle of the South Island, gateway to the lakes and Mount Cook—were the best of our entire month in New Zealand.

Our second day there was sunny, and Jessica and Jonathan explored the farm. They saw a giant pink pig, baby ducklings, chickens, sheep, deer, and a newborn calf which Jessica named "Star" for the white spot on his forehead. Jessie even got to feed the calf with a large bottle of warm milk. She felt his large rough tongue tickle her hand and decided she'd become a vet for big farm animals.

Sonia's teenage daughters took Jonathan for a ride on their mini-tractor, and even let him drive. He touched the metal shepherd's crook used for the sheep and wished to be a farmer. It would soon be lambing season, and Sonia told me about the hard work of lambing and the possible hazards if the weather turned cold.

"Sometimes a ewe carries a rotten lamb, and it's born dead," Sonia said. "Though we scan the sheep (with ultrasound) and separate the ones with twins for special feeding, we cannot tell if the lambs will turn out right. Sometimes the sheep have trouble giving birth because the lamb is turned the wrong way. And if the lambs are born before winter is truly over, a sudden cold spell will kill them. It's sad to see mounds of dead lambs in the middle of the pastures."

For a moment I thought of my own lost babies...

As appealing as South Island farming life seemed, it had its long work hours and its own grief. Sonia looked tired as we chatted while she hung her clean clothes on the line. Her back yard, which was bordered by the stream and cedar trees, had a nice lawn and herb garden. Jessie and Jonathan had met her youngest child, ten-year-old Jessica, and the three of them were jumping on the large trampoline set into the ground.

I looked at Sonia and noticed the fine lines at the corner of her eyes. She rose early and worked late, tending the sheep and her children, and cooking her meals from scratch.

Every morning at 8:30 we could hear her husband Ian starting up the big tractor to bring hay to the animals in the far pastures. For a few days we didn't even meet Ian, but we heard his voice yelling at the barking sheepdogs (their kennels were near our cottage). One evening I called to him across the farmyard, seeing his silhouette in the semidarkness as I asked him to send the children home from the trampoline. He called back to me that he would, and when he went to fetch them, he said,

"Your Mum wants you for tea."

Jessica and Jonathan looked perplexed, not realizing that "tea" could also mean the evening meal.

"We don't have tea very much," Jessica said.

"But our Mom does," Jonathan added.

Then Ian looked perplexed.

꒛

When we did finally meet Ian in daylight, he was a tall man of Irish descent, with blondish hair, thick eyebrows, and blue eyes. His face was a little wrinkled around the edges, from many hours in the wind, snow, and sun.

One afternoon Edd almost drove over a tall rock that had a brass plate on it, and we later found out that was Ian's father's headstone, newly made by Ian himself. Ian had lost his father within the year, and Sonia's father had died of cancer not long before.

Strange how, even in the vast middle of New Zealand's South Island, where you can drive on open roads for hours and not see another car, and where the great lakes and mountains have no cities built upon them, you can come across cancer.

☙

One day we drove west across snowy Burkes Pass where there was a graveyard for the district founders and those killed climbing Mount Cook. We kept driving, past more snowy mountains, to Lake Tekapo. Its whitish-blue glacial water was surrounded by forests and the snowy Southern Alps. A tourist village was built on the end by the dam, and we got out to shop and find hot tea (as usual, we had brought our own snacks with us). We took the path to the lake and found a statue dedicated to sheepdogs, which Jonathan promptly climbed. Then we spied the little stone Church of the Good Shepherd, where a Scottish wedding was taking place. I snapped a photo of a man in a kilt, standing in front of the church.

We drove further westward, through miles of brown high desert, amazed at how quickly the scenery changed. Finally we came to Lake Pukaki, the most beautiful lake we had ever seen. It was larger than Lake Tekapo, a deeper blue, and surrounded by the glacial mountains that led to the highest one in New Zealand, Mount Cook.

We stopped at Lake Pukaki, which had very rocky shores and no village. The day had started out clear, and we could see Mount Cook on the far side of the lake. As afternoon came, clouds descended and covered the mountain's face. We went to the small Tourist Information Center and saw a photo of Mount Cook with no clouds covering it—just sunlight shining broadly on its angled peak. We asked a tourist from England to take our family photo on the banks of Lake Pukaki, our faces smiling against the incredible background of mountains, trees, water, and stones. We got back in the little white rental car and drove the long road that wound along the western bank of Lake Pukaki to Mount Cook.

We passed several streams, forests, and bridges as we climbed higher through a long valley bordered by glacial mountains.

Mount Cook is also called Aoraki, the name of the tallest Maori warrior whose face rises into clouds. Mount Cook is covered by glaciers 100 feet thick, year round, that flow down on all sides to valleys or seashore. People walk on those glaciers with spiked boots, but the danger of an unseen crevasse can kill the most experienced climber. The Maori say that to walk upon the snowy face of Mount Aoraki is to violate his dignity.

The tallest peak in New Zealand, Mount Cook towers 12,000 feet above a valley that is ringed by other members of The Southern Alps. Dozens of glaciers cut through the mountains, moraines line their jagged sides, and streams and rivers pour down to Lake Pukaki, stretching for miles and ringed by mountains on 3 sides.

I had never seen such amazing geology. Edd watched good-humoredly as I snapped photo after photo. At the end of the road was Mount Cook Village were we visited the Tourist Information Center, the Hermitage Hotel, and then hiked toward Kea Point, hoping to see one of the rare alpine parrots we had bought a books and postcards about.

"Keeeaaa!" Jessie called as she held out her arm. I hoped large, green-gray wings centered with orange would descend from the cliffs above us. But Jessie's call only echoed through the gorge. She kept her eyes skyward, searching. Finally she lowered her arm and her gaze. This was our last day in the mountains and our last chance to see a Kea.

"Oh, well," I said, putting my arm across her shoulders. "That means we'll have to come back to New Zealand."

She looked up at me, half hopeful, missing her own little parrot whom we could not bring with us.

Jonathan found a blackbird under a bush, and we saw a hawk in a clearing, eating his dinner. Clouds had already covered all but Mount Cook's lowest cliffs and were heading toward us as a chill wind blew down from the glaciers where—on a clear day—ski planes and helicopters drop off rock climbers, glacier walkers, and brave skiers who glide all the way down to the valley.

❧

After Mount Cook, we drove to Twizel, a desert town near three large brown hills where major battle scenes were filmed for The Lord of the Rings movies. The town seemed lonely and abandoned since the film crews left, though the owners of the film shop told us stories about how the actors would walk in looking like wranglers.

"We saw Aragorn," the man behind the counter told us. "Though we didn't know who he was at the time. He looked completely different when he was all dressed up for battle on horseback. You know, they had to take photos of the actors every day and develop them here, to make sure they looked the same for each shooting."

"Too bad you couldn't keep some of that film," I said wistfully. "What a treasure that would have been."

While Edd and the kids shopped at the market, I walked into The National Bank and was amazed to see it all covered with daffodils. Daffodil chains hung beneath the ceiling. Daffodil flowers filled vases, paper daffodils stuck to teller windows, and little bronze daffodil pins lined a black velvet pad. They even had daffodil pinwheel toys for children.

"Why, you're the Daffodil Bank," I announced to the teller. "Yes, we are one of the big sponsors for Daffodil Day—National Cancer Survivor Day—which is August 29."

"We in America could learn from you. It's not nearly as big a deal over there when the daffodils first bloom in March," I replied.

She smiled and handed me a silk daffodil pin along with the New Zealand money I was exchanging for my travelers' checks. "Everyone in New Zealand buys daffodil pins on Daffodil

Day," she said. "Volunteers get dressed up as Daffodil Fairies and Daffodil Princesses and Daffodil Clowns, and they stand on streetcorners all over the country to help raise an amazing amount of money in one day. It all goes toward cancer research and patient care."

"I'm a cancer survivor and a writer," I informed her, handing her my card.

"Rose over at the Lotto store is our local Cancer Society representative," she informed me. "I'll bet she'd be glad to meet you and get a copy of your book."

"Good idea. Thanks." As I walked out of the bank, I began planning:

Maybe I could go to the National Cancer Society in Auckland when we fly back there before leaving for America, and give them my book...

(And so I did. Edd drove through harrowing traffic to find the Auckland Domain Cancer Society on August 29, and we got a royal reception. A staff member named Marin showed us the new live-in facility complete with private apartments, community kitchen, library, and rooftop garden—and a shop full of daffodil items, where I would buy a pair of enamel daffodil earrings for $1.00, and we would pose for our family photo, each wearing a daffodil pin...)

I went to the car to get one of my little blue books with the photo of me a year after the chemo treatments, when my hair was as short and curly as two-year-old Jonathan's. He clung to my back in a baby pack while Jessie, only five, stood at my side as we paused beside an evergreen tree while hiking in Canada...

Rose at the Lotto Store seemed happy to get the book. She smiled and recommended that I check out the Cancer Society in Christchurch too.

"Did you know that a river runs through Christchurch, and it has old buildings and trees like an English university town?" Rose asked. She was an enthusiastic woman with bright red hair and a green sweater.

"I heard it was pretty."

"There are willows and black swans by the river, and you can push a wooden boat on it, and there are stone bridges arcing over it. And in a park by the river stands a twisted piece of metal from The World Trade Center in New York, to remind us of what happened on September 11, 2001."

"Wow!" I replied (since Twizel was not busy, one could carry on long conversations in places of business).

"Also, you could contact the local Cancer Society Representative," Rose added, handing me a card with a woman's name on it.

If only people in America were as enthusiastic about my books...

∽

The night before we had to leave Possum Cottage, we took Ian and Sonia out to dinner at the old hotel in town. We were the only customers there that rainy night, and we ate by the bar near a fireplace and candles. The meal was good—hot fresh fish and beef with roasted potatoes and salads.

"I come from a farm in the next valley," Sonia told us. "My family has been in New Zealand for generations. Ian's father helped him start our present farm, and we had to clear it all of gorse plants. What a work that was, digging out the roots with tractors."

"Aye, our great-grandparents were some of the first settlers in this area," Ian added.

After dinner, I gave Sonia a copy of <u>Crossing the Chemo Room</u>. Ian remarked that I was a year too late. Edd and I shared our cancer survival story anyway. Sonia and Ian leaned toward us across the table, their faces beautiful in the candlelight as they listened to our words about how Christ's love—The Light of the World—can bring us through the darkest places.

In the long silence that followed, while we ate our dessert, I remembered another kind of darkness when Ian asked, "What did you think about Albury?"

He was referring to a village we had visited a couple of days ago. We were actually looking at houses for sale in the general area (with the dream of buying one and moving to New Zealand). Albury's prices were cheap, but Ian and Sonia had told us why.

"The village is dying out. Many people have sold their houses and moved, and those who stay and rent are migrant workers passing through," Ian had warned us.

"The shops have closed," Sonia added. "Only the school and pub stay open. And that part of the valley is dark and cold in winter."

We went to the town anyway. It was in a low part of the valley, near a river ford. As we drove past its empty streets, we noticed three old churches—stone, brick, and wood—that were not being used. One was even boarded up. Yet in the pub window was an advertisement for an occult fair at a local farm.

We drove slowly, looking for the listed house which turned out to be a charming white wood place with hedges around a grassy yard. The renters spotted us and walked toward our car.

"What are you doing?" the woman asked.

"Just out looking at houses," Edd replied cheerfully.

"The owner's given us to the end of the month," the woman replied in a scruffy voice. The man only stared.

They were a strange middle-aged couple with the look of drug addicts or alcoholics. Something in their blank eyes seemed menacing as they asked where we were staying. The man had paint smeared on his shirt, and the woman leaned toward me, over the partly-opened car window, her straggly brown-gray hair hanging in her eyes. For a moment I thought of my wild Gypsy heritage and wondered if the woman read people's palms.

"Are you from America?" she asked.

"Yes," I replied, pulling back from the window.

"Well, the owner told us the house has been sold!" she declared.

"Then we'll be going," Edd decided, putting the car in gear.

As we drove back toward Possum Cottage, we saw a lone teenage boy walking on the highway, toward the abandoned town. He looked bored and depressed, and we wished one of those churches was playing Christian rock music and blazing with light...

⁂

"Oh, you were right about that town," Edd replied as he sipped his coffee. "Perhaps you could keep your eyes open for something for sale closer to our sheep farm."

Sonia promised she would. Ian offered us a parting drink, and we left the cheerful hotel pub and stepped into the night.

Wind buffeted the car, and rain poured down heavily as Ian drove us back to the farm. He invited us into the farmhouse, and I was amazed at their huge kitchen filled with jars of cooking essentials I probably couldn't put a name to. Sonia offered us tea, but I could tell they were tired, so we declined. But before we left, I took out my green laser light. As we all stood on their porch, I shone it upward through the rain and trees.

"Astronomers use these to point out the stars," I said in a hushed tone.

"Well, look at that!" Ian exclaimed as he watched the bright green laser which seemed to reach for miles, sparkling with raindrops.

We all stood, Kiwis and Americans, children and adults, awed at the simple power of light.

As Edd, the kids, and I walked back toward Possum Cottage with borrowed umbrellas and calls of "good night," I realized I had just impressed a stoic New Zealand farmer.

⁂

The next morning, both Ian and Sonia came to the cottage yard to say goodbye.

"When you come back, I'll take you up the Rangitata River in my jet boat," Ian offered as he leaned on a fencepost.

"That would be great!" I replied.

"And thanks for the dinner and company last night," Sonia added gently. "I will read your book and send you an email."

"Maybe next time I could help around the farm," Edd offered. "I like to chop wood."

"Well, there's always need for that," Ian laughed.

※

Before we left Possum Cottage to drive to Christchurch and fly back to Auckland, we took special care to leave the cottage in good shape, saving Sonia some work. I matched up all the china, arranged the knickknacks in order, and stacked the books neatly.

As I packed what was left of my books, I thought about the people we had met, to whom I had given my card or a book: the Auckland rental car lady who said "no worries"; the waitress from the Taupo cafe; Terri, the Mum from Hastings; the River Man from the great Waikato; the Internet Cafe computer whiz; the Grandmother skier from Mount Ruapehu; Liz and her daughters from Wellington; Pastor Danny of the Anglican Church; Pete, the South Island Cowboy; the Mountain Bartender with a Hangover; the Australian Barmaid who shattered a tray of glasses; the librarians of several libraries; Rose from The Cancer Society in Twizel; the teller at The Daffodil Bank; and Sonia and Ian, our sheepfarm hosts.

Would we see these people again? Surely they had touched our lives as much as we had touched theirs.

We finished packing our suitcases, filled with New Zealand items like tea, chocolate, honey, postcards, maps, books, and toys. I even had a walking stick made from the Lance tree, which looks like a brace of sharp-edged weapons as a juvenile tree and like a normal tree as an adult. On the top of the walking stick was a two-cent coin, etched with the yellow Kowhai flowers and a fern.

I had finally found my own silver fern pin, like the one Liz wore on the day she took us around Wellington. I wore it on my black sweater in remembrance of our amazing month.

"I want to stay and live in New Zealand," Jessica announced, looking toward the fields of animals. "I could have my own horse."

"And I could learn to ski," Jonathan added as he stared at the mountains.

"And I could golf and be a farmer," Edd dreamed.

"And I could explore the lakes and glaciers and write about them," I declared.

As we drove down Ian and Sonia's tree-lined driveway, we noticed the daffodils blooming beside the road, against a patch of grass. The first sunlight of spring shone through evergreen boughs and onto the yellow flowers.

And for the rest of our stay in New Zealand and when we returned to California, we told everyone,

"We left our hearts in the Land of the Silver Fern."

California Burning

*"Lord, by Your favor,
You have made
my mountain stand strong."*
Psalm 30:7

"I don't want to die!" Jessica screamed as she glanced over her right shoulder, out the car's rear window.

A wall of flames was lapping up the darkness of our mountainside, heading for the Rim.

"Oh my gosh," Jonathan uttered. "See how high the fire is!"

I kept looking back while trying to keep the car on the narrow highway. When I got a chance, I pulled over into a turnout to watch. The crimson flames seemed beautiful, alluring, and destructive.

"Don't stop!" Jessie yelled. "And don't you dare take a picture! We should have left seven hours ago."

"Don't worry. We're safe. We'll get down the mountain," I tried to assure her. She held a big white bird cage on her lap with a parakeet in it. Penny the Parrot was in the other bird cage, back beside Jonathan. Bubbles the Beta Fish was in his little evacuation bowl in the car's cupholder.

"I want Daddy!" Jessie whined as I took one last look at the approaching wall of fire before merging with the long line of headlights making a slow, orderly caravan down the burning mountain.

Jess is a helpful, quiet, intelligent soul who is gentle with birds and people. When it comes to catastrophes, she scares easily—like her parrot who flies off my shoulder if startled by the ceiling fan.

"You can call Daddy on the cell phone," I suggested. "Tell him the fire is getting closer, the traffic is bad, and he should leave now."

Edd had stayed behind for last-minute house checks and to load up the three cats.

"Do you think Midnight will be afraid?" Jess asked, sounding calmer as she dialed on my small red phone.

"She'll be safe in her carry box," I replied.

Jess spoke briefly with Edd who assured her he would be leaving soon—especially if people stopped calling him on the phone.

We drove through another mountain town, and I wondered if my friend Mary Pat, who had to evacuate a couple of months ago, would be leaving her home again. We entered the lower highway which cut quickly down toward the valley, only to see flames leaping up from the valley floor almost to the top, parallel to the highway.

"Oh my gosh," Jonathan said again, pointing in the darkness toward the car's right side.

"Jessie, call Daddy one more time. Tell him a wall of flame is is closing in on the highway from the west, and he'd better hurry. The fire can't be more than a mile away. They'll shut this evacuation route soon, and it'll take him five hours to get down the mountain the back way."

I tried to control the alarm in my voice, my mind wandering as I drove down near the line of fire. I found myself thinking about my lost parents and brother, about going through cancer, about the miscarriages. Surely my family and I would survive this wildfire...

Jessie got her message through just as Edd was leaving.

"I'm scared," she admitted as she set the cellphone down.

An eerie red light danced on her right cheek, her arm, and down her long braid. "I don't want to die so young, like this, on a burning mountain."

"There are a lot of firefighters up here," I assured her. "Remember how we kept checking the fire's progress by driving down to the lookout point? When the fire got close is when we decided to leave. No one even told us to go! We had all day to pack the stuff we needed. Now that area will be packed with fire engines, but the planes won't be able to dump water after dark."

"Will our house burn?" she asked, staring at me in the dark car, the birthmark on her left cheek barely visible in the dashboard's green light.

"I don't know," I replied, knowing that something would be burning.

As we drove lower toward the valley, strange white flashes spread across the mountain like lightning.

"What's that?" Jessie asked.

"I think those are electrical transformers exploding."

◈

My mind started wandering back to earlier that evening. The electricity had gone out right before we evacuated. We had to wear headlamps to carry bags down our stairs. We swept the beams through each room one last time, wondering what final item to take, what we wouldn't want to burn. We grabbed a few more framed photographs and kids' toys, then stepped outside to a quiet street with no lamps shining from the windows of already-abandoned homes.

◈

Oh please protect the mountain, I prayed as I tried to keep from crying while entering the valley freeway and leaving our home behind.

Over an hour later, we arrived at our friends the Connelley's, in the desert valley. As soon as we got out of the car, Heidi remarked,

"You smell like smoke."

I nodded and replied, "You helped me survive cancer seven

years ago, and now you keep me from the fire."

I practically fell into her arms.

Jessica and Jonathan ran to play with Heidi's children and their cousin Linda, whom Heidi and her husband Jonathan had adopted. Big Jonathan helped us unload birdcages, suitcases, and toys. We got situated in our temporary shelter as Edd pulled up in a car full of boxes and cats.

"I got down just before they closed the highway," he told me, kissing me in the dark by his car. "I heard the fire jumped the upper highway and was coming up the mountaintop."

If it continued, it would reach our house ...

We turned on the news and watched updates of the fire's progress—for the next five harrowing days: in the middle of the night when we couldn't sleep, in the early morning when our nightmares woke us, in the afternoon when we felt helpless because we couldn't go see for ourselves, in the evening after dinner when we tried to talk about something else but faltered.

Sometimes it looked as though the firefighters would succeed at keeping the flames from jumping the highway to the dead treetops and communities of homes and businesses, schools and churches, that lined the top of the mountains from the west to the eastern heights. Other times the flames broke free and burned homes and businesses.

We watched as towering flames licked along a large, familiar A-frame roof. The news helicopter announcer told us it was historic Wylie Woods Presbyterian Conference Center—where just two weeks ago the kids and I had taken a Homeschool Tree class taught by Doris Bowers. And then, late on Wednesday night, October 29, the flames burned back toward Lake Arrowhead and consumed the community of Cedar Glen.

We had friends there. The red log cabin where Doris lived—had it been lost? And the garage, stacked full of teaching material collected over 40 years, was it reduced to ashes? Had she rescued anything in her old camper truck? Had she evacuated? She would be the type to stay until the last possible moment, keeping watch.

And what about Clayton and Jessica Connolly, who got

married last April? He is a musician, leading worship with Edd at Calvary Chapel and teaching children how to play the piano. Had all his keyboards melted? And Jessica, the oceanographer, were her college textbooks and shell collections gone? Had their photos and their wedding presents burned?

And Suzanne Bowen, who owns the local health food store and has five children. Had her house been swept away? And all those toys and homeschool books and bottles of herbal remedies?

☙

A fireman pulled a T.V. newscrew from their burning van when flames arced over both sides of Rim highway. Veteran fire captains said they had seen nothing like this fire that hit the tall, dead pines above one neighborhood. Years of drought, bark beetles, hot weather, and Santa Anna winds caused Three-hundred-foot flames that shot into the air like tornados swirling with sparks. Sap-filled trees exploded, shooting burning branches like missiles toward new fires. Rooftops crashed like flying saucers. Propane tanks blew up one after the other, and open gas pipes burned long after the fire swept through like The Perfect Storm.

"It's just like the dream that woke me up on Saturday morning, two hours before an arsonist lit our mountain on fire," I moaned to Heidi and her children gathered around the T.V. screen. "And Edd looked out our kitchen window and, for a moment in the sunrise, saw flames above the trees. Without debate, we started packing.

"And out the window was a calm fall day, with the sun shining, a breeze blowing the cedar branches, and the maple trees turning red and orange. And we wandered around our mountain home—like a treehouse in Lothlorian—with its big windows and heavy French doors and honey-colored paneling—and all the paintings, and the rock fireplace with photos on the mantel—and wondered if it all would burn.

"And we walked out onto the deck and stared at the dry

stream by the yard and the forest backed up against us, dust and pine needles and fallen leaves everywhere—and saw only fuel...

"And I sent an email from my computer room, to all the people on my Mailing List:

"'We Are Evacuating.'

"And Doyle and Paula Eden, friends who live closer to the fire, were watching a movie when they checked their email. They hadn't even known the fire was racing up the slopes toward them, at the rate of an acre a minute.

"No one told us to leave."

Heidi, with her long reddish hair and practical voice, stated,

"Well, that just shows that when the fire gets close, you go."

And I wanted to laugh at her statement, but I couldn't. We kept watching the news.

"The heat was so great that it knocked me on my back," a news photographer said. "If I had not been wearing this yellow fireman's jacket, I would have been burned."

"I can't talk about it," said a longtime newscaster who had stayed up all night, reporting. His white shirt was singed with black spots, and ash made his hair look gray. "I just feel for all these people who have lost their homes."

And an anchorman wailed,

"The Crown Jewel of California is burning!"

And we, safe in Heidi's living room, could only watch the drama and pray for rain. We also watched the fire in her fireplace, orange and red and white and yellow flames flowing together, dancing like something alive, licking along the wood and sending sparks up the chimney. Seductive, warm, and romantic, fire can save lives or destroy them. Would some of the sparks escape and lodge in the trees or rooftops?

Frustrated with the T.V. stations that kept getting the mountain names wrong, we turned to the Internet and Ranger Al's accurate accounts on his website. Al, who stayed on the mountain to help the firefighters, listed the streets and houses that burned—a document of several pages.

We checked our email, hoping to hear from mountain friends like Josh and Lisa Williams, with whom we had dinner a week before the fire. Ironically, Edd and I had complained to them about our difficult October! Lisa, who used to be a radio host, sent us emails. Josh, a high-tech computer guy, kept in touch by cellphone. Even Pastor Tom from Calvary Chapel made a list of all the cellphone owners in our evacuated church, and he called to check on us.

"I feel like a shepherd with all the flock gone," he said over the static-filled receiver.

And friends from all over the country, Ireland, and New Zealand sent us emails with offered prayers.

We were dispersed to the valleys and cities and beaches, in Red Cross Shelters, houses, or hotels, but we kept together electronically and hoped to return home soon.

Even our evacuation areas were not safe. A fire broke out near the wine country. We nervously watched the southeast flames crest distant hills, then got out binoculars and followed low-flying planes as they dropped water. Further south, much of San Diego burned. People were killed in their cars while trying to flee the fires in their suburban neighborhoods. And in the northwest counties, houses and canyons burned. Smoke rose in giant, mushroom plumes in all directions. Horizons glowed red, and the air was heavy with ash.

"Is it the end of the world?" Jonathan asked as he climbed up to watch beside me on a hill of rocks.

"Not yet," I assured him, tousling his curly hair.

"I wish we were still in New Zealand," he whimpered. "Where there are lakes and rivers. Remember how you dressed me in my Frodo costume and took my picture in a field?"

"Yes, I remember. And we drove to Mount Cook and saw the snow and glaciers, in the Land of the Lord of the Rings."

୶

And so, like a scene from a film, much of Southern California burned that week—the largest fire in United States history. Thousands of acres burned, 3500 homes perished—whole suburbs together, entire country towns wiped out. Several people lost their lives, including a fireman who died protecting a stranger's property.

And then, amazingly, the weather changed. The Santa Anna winds died down, and the breezes blew in westerly, over the cool Pacific Ocean. Rain swept down from Alaska, water muddied ashes in the valleys, and snow dusted our mountains. That was not in the T.V. weather forecast. When was the last time we had snow in October?

∽

Two weeks after evacuation, we drove up a burned mountain. A full moon shone above short black stubs that dotted the canyons. Bare black treetrunks shone eerily in the moonlight, and even the dirt and rocks were ashen. And we thought,

Our mountain looks like Mordor.

∽

Everyone we knew in one neighborhood lost homes, except for Doris Bowers whose house was high enough atop a hill that the flames did not reach it. Even people from the local newspaper where I work were hit, including my Editor Davey Porter, my friend Laura who works in advertising, and Gordon who does the fishing column.

I wandered down to that burned-out neighborhood, dazed, to take some photographs and write a story for the paper:

There is a bridge between 2 houses, on the corner of Hook Creek and Bridge Roads. The house to the right looks ready for a fall day, its cheerful redwood walls and scalloped roof surrounded by green bushes, a lawn, and the red and yellow leaves of healthy trees. A brooke bubbles at its verge, under the bridge. The house to the left is the last one burned in a long line of devastation. Everything is gray and black: car shells, twisted metal, broken steps, heaps of ash. Charred stone chimneys rise like memorials in what used to be a neighborhood.

Here the firemen took a stand in the worst firestorm in California history, where 300-foot flames burned tall dead pine trees which exploded like bombs.

Further down Hook Creek Road lies the ruins of another house, the home of newlyweds Clayton and Jessica Connolly of Calvary Chapel. Clayton, a worship leader, rescued his keyboards and wedding photos, but little else. When a CNN television news crew found him standing next to his leveled house, they asked why he was smiling.

Clayton replied, "They can take my home, my property, and even my wedding gifts, but they can't take my Jesus."

Up near The Malt Shop, a red log cabin survived. Its owner, Doris Bowers, has lived in these mountains for 40 years. She is a homeschool science teacher, and all of her teaching materials are stored in her garage. As she gratefully checked on her property, she said,

"Well, at least we have some trees left on this mountain. Fewer to cut down now."

Then she got in her truck, waved, and headed down the mountain to teach another class.

And other people showed their gratitude for surviving the fire. On the lawn of one untouched house a handpainted sign read "Thank you. We love you all, and so does Jesus." A big American flag waved over a burnt house further down the way. On a slope, someone sat in a white tent on the remains of his home. At the old Car Wash, a Fire Rescue Center began offering counseling, hot meals, clothes, and all types of necessary aid. Utility trucks and repair crews lined the roads.

The neighborhood is already rebuilding. Maybe it was never really lost, for the people who lived there survived. And the rest of us, hardy mountain people who knew the risks when we moved into the forest, share the experience with each other at the grocery store or in the post office. We ask where we evacuated to and talk about the fire. Sometimes we cry into comforting arms. And perhaps we remember a verse from Psalm 30:

"Lord, by Your favor You have made my mountain stand strong."

And so, like the Bible verse suggested, much of our mountain survived though 100,000 acres, 1000 homes, and 10 businesses burned. On a map put out by the Crest Forest Fire Department (www.cffd.org), the fire area looked like a giant, open red hand grasping the mountaintop on three sides. Their website's slide show, photographs taken mostly by firefighters, gave us a glimpse of the monster they fought. Yet on most of the Rim you could not tell there had been a wildfire, as our house and many others stood untouched and did not even smell of smoke. Thank you God, for changing the weather. And thank you, firefighters, for taking a stand at Strawberry Peak, a mile from our home, where 1200 of you lined up with shovels. Like Gandalf with the fiery monster, you stood at a point, dug in your staff, and said,

"You shall not pass."

"Return of the King"

Christmas, 2003

It's Christmas again. Our house on the mountain, safe from the October fires, is lit with tiny colored lights. New snow dusts the evergreen trees, and you would never know how dry everything was two months ago and that, through satellite T.V., the whole world watched our mountain burn.

Jessica is upstairs vacuuming, singing Christmas carols above the machine's hum. Edd and Jonathan are at church, practicing with the musicians for our Candlelight Service. Kristen is in San Diego with her new husband Jeremy, enjoying their first Christmas together. Ryan is with his dad and stepmom, on their sailboat in the bay.

A longtime friend of mine, a photographer named Brad Human, died last month of a heart attack. He gave me my first writing job, doing brochures for Beverly Hills homes. He did the photos, and I wrote descriptive words like "ambiance." He and his wife Gladi ended up homeschooling their children, and he became a portrait-taker. He took Jessica and Jonathan's homeschool photos since they were in kindergarten, down in the valley and up here on the mountain.

Now he sees more than a camera ever captured.

My cousin Larry lost his ex-wife to ovarian cancer a few weeks ago. Though they had divorced, he still cared for her. He sent me a pretty notecard, telling me the recent news, his words all brokenhearted.

"I'm taking time off from work," he wrote. "I'll visit my

parents and then travel for a few months. I'm doing as well as can be expected."

I hope he ends up on our mountain. The kids have never met him. I hope he finds new life.

A certain friend and I have not spoken since the fire evacuation. She thought everyone was in "mass hysteria" and didn't need to leave. She said she'd wait until the sheriff came knocking on her door to mandate her departure. And why did the school cancel its Halloween Party?

I felt angry at her selfishness, for I had seen those flames sweep up the mountainside toward people's homes. No one told us to leave. And when we returned, I felt like taking her for a walk through a charred neighborhood, where all the houses burned—to show her "mass hysteria."

"I've evacuated three times now," she emailed me. "I'm tired."

So are the rest of us, I thought. What have you done to help the fire victims?

A woman from church committed suicide last week. I had talked to her only a few times. She read my <u>Chemo</u> book. She had tried to end her life before, and she told me once that she was a cancer survivor, too, and the cancer had returned, and she couldn't face it, and she felt compelled to give up. She had endured an abusive childhood and difficult adult life, filled with emotional and physical pain.

"But think of your husband and children," I replied. "Your teenage daughter is lovely. Do you realize that she wears her hair like you, pulled back in a clip? And your youngest is only five."

She wept in reply. I hugged her, and she trembled in my arms—like Lori, who was dying of lung cancer when I embraced her once at Dr. Schinke's office, and it seemed as though our souls touched.

Lori did not want to die so young and leave her daughter.

And this woman from church, did she walk past the family Christmas tree and see all the pretty lights? Did she walk into her children's rooms, one by one, and watch them sleeping in the dim night? Did she see their faces and the rhythm of their breaths? How, then, could she go to the family garage, get in the car, drive to the lookout point above a million lights, and take a bottle of deadly pills? A Highway Patrol man found her body the next morning, slumped over the steering wheel.

But her life did not count for nothing, ending as it did.

She and her husband lost their business in the October fire. Perhaps she is another victim of the flames.

I got a postcard from my old friend Cherie who had her fifth child, the boy to replace the one she lost. She sent a photo from hot Arizona, the kids all wearing short-sleeve shirts, little Buck smiling in her lap. It's been six years since my miscarriage at four months, right before Christmas. Two years since my last miscarriage. I guess I'm getting over all that.

I have an hour before the church's candlelight service begins. Do I take a walk in the starlight, nap, or try to bring all my scattered thoughts together at the ending of my book?

I sprained my shoulder from too much writing and don't feel like mailing any more cards—the ones I designed on the computer, using a photo of Edd, Jessica, Jonathan, and me in our parkas on the snowy summit of Mount Ruapehu. It was winter last August in New Zealand—handy for making Christmas cards in advance.

I still receive email from Rev. Danny in Wellington, my friend Liz, and the Callaghans from the South Island sheep farm. My friend Carol from England sent a Yorkshire calendar, filled with pictures to entice me back.

My heart is more inclined to New Zealand, a new country like America but without Hollywood and all the hype. I'm glad that Peter Jackson proved that you don't have to live in L.A. to make some great movies.

Sunday we dressed up in capes and went to our little mountain theater to see the final <u>Lord of the Rings</u> movie, <u>The Return of the King</u>.

We pointed out places we recognized—Mount Cook with its glaciers, the three brown hills near Twizel, the fern forests of Taupo, the Rangitata River and its plains. And we wanted to return to the Land of the Silver Fern.

I identified with Eowyn, the shieldmaiden of Rohan who dressed up in armor and fought with the men. She cut off the head of a dragon and slayed its Black Rider. And a great battle was fought, and Frodo couldn't toss the ring into the molten fire of Mount Doom, even after the long journey and all the help of his friends. An enemy snatched the ring from his finger and fell with it into the fire, destroying the Dark Lord and his forces.

Aragorn became King. He exchanged his motley Ranger look for a golden crown. Arwen renounced her elvish life to become his mortal wife. And Frodo, who bore the burden of the evil ring—to the point of exhaustion, pain, and the end of hope—lay beside faithful Sam on a rock in the midst of a red lava sea. Though eagles rescued him, elves refreshed him, and he returned to the peaceful Shire, Frodo could not stay with his Hobbit friends. The pain in his shoulder—caused by a Nazgul blade—never healed.

After a great adventure, it is hard to live a normal life.

Jonathan, sitting in front of me in his green cape clasped by a leaf pin, his glow-in-the-dark sword by his side, wept at the movie's end when Frodo sailed off with the elves, into the western light.

Christmas is a time for lights. Jesus came

"To give light to those
who sit in darkness
and the shadow of death,
To guide our feet
into the way of peace." (Luke 1:79)

And Jesus told those who follow Him:

"You are the light of the world.
A city that is set on a hill
cannot be hidden.
Nor do they light a lamp
and put it under a basket,
but on a lampstand,

and it gives light to all
who are in the house." (Matthew 5:14 & 15)

In Jesus' time, there was no electric light. All was flame, real and burning, with power to save or destroy.

When I see the vast valleys of electric lights spreading toward the ocean, I can hardly believe I live in one of the most populated places of the world. Our mountaintop holds small towns hidden behind the rim, among the trees and clouds. When the slopes and peaks were aflame, all eyes were drawn to the sight.

May it ever blaze with light, as when Pippin lit the bonfire of Gondor, and all the mountaintops burned with answering signals, ridge to ridge, the flames beautiful against snow, to the hilltop of Rohan—a call to fight.

Resources

Internet Sources

1. The American Cancer Society—http://www.cancer.org or call 1-800-ACS-2345

Here you can find all kinds of information on cancer events and late-breaking research news, treatment, support, volunteering to help cancer patients, local ACS chapters in your area, etc.. Also, you can call and speak to a nurse and order informative booklets.

2. Cancer Society of New Zealand—http://www.cancernz.org.nz

This site's logo is a daffodil, and Daffodil Day in New Zealand is an amazing fundraising event where almost all Kiwis buy silk daffodil pins to support cancer research and patient care. Helpful information and support, too. Americans could learn much from this organization.

3. The National Cancer Institute's CancerNet—http://cancernet.nci.nih.gov
or call 1-800-4-CANCER

This is the best technical cancer source on the Internet—home of the famous PDQ ("Physicians Data Query"—information written for either doctors or patients). Find all about the latest research, types of cancer, treatment, recovery, etc.

4. Oncolink (Univ. of Penn. Cancer Center)—http://cancer.med.upenn.edu

Check out the survivor stories, artwork, photos, support groups, technical information, links to other cancer sites, etc.

5. Steve Dunn's Cancerguide—http://cancerguide.org
Very helpful for patients—survival stories, tips on how to research cancer, lots of Internet links, etc.

6. City of Hope—http://cityofhope.org

Get the latest cancer research information, find out about bone marrow transplantation, and read "bmt" survivor stories (complete with photos). You can also learn about volunteer opportunities, especially the annual "Walk for Hope" against breast cancer.

7. "True Life Stories"—http://www.true-life.org.uk

Not a cancer site, this is a Christian e-zine out of England that publishes stories about people all over the world who found God's help during traumatic life events. Cool graphics, easy to read.

8. Lonna Williams' Website
—http://www.lonnawilliams.com

Browse through excerpts from my yet unpublished children's stories, <u>Like a Tree Planted</u>, <u>Crossing the Chemo Room</u>, and <u>Selah of the Summit</u>. See the silly photos I got friends and family members to pose for. Check out my landscapes of England, Canada, California, and Ireland. Read my interviews of top figure skaters and articles on "Lord of the Rings and Harry Potter," cancer survival tips, and homeschooling.

9. The Susan G. Komen Foundation
—http://www.komen.org
or call (800) I'M AWARE (462-9273)

A user-friendly site where you can read survivor stories and find out what the Susan G. Komen Foundation is doing to help fight breast cancer. You can see a list of national and local activities such as "Race for the Cure." You can find out more about breast cancer, post your own survival story, or order a cute pink ribbon pin.

10. Focus on the Family—http://www.family.org

Dr. Dobson's family-oriented website that features up-to-date film and book reviews as well as articles on social topics. Great resources and support for children, teens, women, and men. Includes a section on miscarriage loss.

11. The Tolkien Forum—http://www.thetolkienforum.com

My favorite J.R.R. Tolkien website—well designed, organized, and maintained. It has the latest Peter Jackson <u>Lord of the Rings</u> film information as well as scholarly histories and languages of Middle-earth. On its many forums, you can post ideas, original poetry, and observations on anything related to hobbits, elves, etc.

12. A Quiet Refuge—http://www.quietrefuge.com

A website dedicated to parents who have had miscarriages or lost young children, made by parents who experienced the same. It has a section for making an album to remember your child, help with the grieving process, and a calm, soothing design. Russ and June Gordon's mission statement is: "In

Matthew 18:10, Jesus is speaking to a gathered crowd. He pulls a little child close to him and says, 'See that you do not look down upon one of these little ones. For I tell you that their angels in heaven always see the face of my Father in heaven.' We believe that children, even unborn children, are very special to God. We should value them as He does." You can email Russ and June Gordon from their website.

13. Pregnancy Loss Info—http://www.pregnancyloss.info

A beautiful, touching site with calm music and good photos, by Deanna Roy, who had a miscarriage at 20 weeks and later lost a twin. She has great links to helpful sources, medical information for those going through a miscarriage or who have had one, emotional support, religious questions, other women's stories, a teen section, helpful books, music, and artwork, and just about everything you could think of in regards to getting support during such a difficult time. You can email Deanna from her website.

14. Angels in Heaven—http://www.angelsinheaven.org

Another beautiful, helpful website that is actually a ministry started by Doug and Debbie Heydrick who had their own miscarriage. Their ministry offers counseling, keepsake albums, and keepsake cards. They have many resources and links for those who have had miscarriages. Their theme verse is 2 Corinthians 1:3&4: "Praise be to the God and Father of our Lord Jesus Christ, Father of compassion and the God of all comfort, who comforts us in all our troubles, so that we can comfort those in any trouble with the comfort we ourselves have received from God." You can email Doug and Debbie from their website.

15. The Compassionate Friends—http://www.compassionatefriends.org

This website assists families "toward the positive resolution of grief following the death of a child of any age and to provide information to help others be supportive. The Compassionate Friends is a national nonprofit, self-help support organization that offers friendship and understanding to bereaved parents, grandparents, and siblings. There is no religious affiliation, and there are no membership dues or fees. The secret of TCF's success is simple: As seasoned grievers reach out to the newly bereaved, energy that has been directed inward begins to flow outward, and both are helped to heal." My friend Marilyn Heavilin, who wrote <u>Roses in December</u>, got involved in this group that began in England in the 1960s. The site offers great links, resources, tools, etc. Click to find chapters in your area or call toll-free (877) 969-0010.

Cancer Booklets

1. <u>A Woman's Guide to Breast Cancer Diagnosis and Treatment</u> by The California Department of Health Services (no date). Order from Breast Cancer Treatment Options, Medical Board of California, 1426 Howe Ave., Suite 54, Sacramento, CA 95825 or FAX requests to (916) 263-2479.

Find out, in this short booklet, about essential breast cancer detection, treatment, and support (with phone numbers, address, and helpful illustrations).

2. <u>Chemotherapy and You</u> by the National Cancer Institute (Publication No. 94-1136), July, 1993.

This booklet explains how basic chemotherapy treatments work, their possible side effects, and precautions you should take while undergoing treatment.

3. <u>Taking Time</u> by the National Cancer Institute (Publication No. 94-2059), December, 1993.

Written for patients, their families, and their friends, this booklet discusses helpful ways to deal with doctors and hospitals, emotional needs, exercise, stress, family issues, self-image, and long-term recovery

Books Related to Cancer and Nutrition

(nearly everything I list can be found on amazon.com)

1. <u>Fighting Cancer</u> by Annette and Richard Bloch. R.A. Bloch Cancer Foundation: Kansas City, MO, 1985.

All sorts of good, practical advice from the co-founder of H & R Block, Inc. Doctors told Mr. Bloch that he should get his affairs in order because he would soon die of terminal lung cancer. He recovered and founded a nonprofit cancer support center at the University of Missouri. Richard also started the famous "PDQ" now on NCI's CancerNet (Internet Homepage).

2. <u>Making the Chemotherapy Decision</u> by David Drum. Lowell House: Los Angeles, 1996.

I wish this book was out when I was first diagnosed. I should have read it before I started chemotherapy. It lists most of the chemo drugs, how they work, side effects, etc. It also tells you what to expect emotionally during and after chemo. Great for patients and their families and friends.

3. <u>It's Always Something</u> by Gilda Radner. Avon Books: New York, 1989.

I really enjoyed this sad, funny, honest book by Gilda, the

well-known comedienne who died of "the most unfunny thing in the world"—ovarian cancer—in 1989. Her narrative is easy to follow and interesting. I wish I had met Gilda. Maybe someday I will.

4. Cancer Combat by Dean and Jessica King and Jonathan Pearlroth. Bantam: New York, 1998.

This book is filled with survivor stories by all sorts of cancer patients and tackles topics from bills to treatments to recovery and support.

5. The Climb of my Life by Laura Evans. Harper: San Francisco, 1996.

A mountaineer chronicles her battle with breast cancer and her founding of "Expedition Inspiration," a group that takes recovering breast cancer patients on mountain climbs.

6. No Mountain Too High by Andrea Gabbard. Seal Press, 1998.

Another hiker and breast cancer patient tells her survival story and how she led a group of breast cancer-recovering women to climb the highest mountain in South America.

7. No Time to Die by Liz Tiberis. Little, Brown & Co.: New York, 1998.

A fashion industry leader chronicles her successful battle with ovarian cancer.

8. Eileen's Story by Rosamond Richardson. Element: Rockport, MA, 1997.

The easy-to-read tale of a woman who had "incurable" lymphoma and recovered.

9. <u>When Life Becomes Precious</u> by Elise Babcock. Bantom Doubleday: New York, 1997.

A guide for loved ones and friends of cancer patients, this book gives stories of patients along with advice on what to say and expect when a loved one (or you) hear the diagnosis of cancer. Elise Babcock is an experienced counselor whose father died of cancer.

10. <u>Portraits of Hope: Conquering Breast Cancer</u>. Text by Marcia Stevens. Photography by Nora Feller. Sherril. The Wonderland Press and Smithmark Publishers: New York, 1998.

A beautiful collection of 52 women's stories about surviving breast cancer. Great photographs. Some of the women are celebrities; some are previously unknown. Easy to read and encouraging.

11. <u>Coping with Cancer</u> by John E. Packo. Christian Publications, Inc.: Camp Hill, PA, 1991.

A minister's story of his battle with lymphoma. He gives Biblical perspectives on suffering and healing.

12. <u>Cancer Lives at Our House</u> by Beatrice Hofman Hoek. Baker Books: Grand Rapids, MI, 1997.

A mother recounts her family's reaction to her breast cancer. She gives helpful advice and Biblical insight on how to help family members and friends of cancer patients.

13. <u>Prescription for Nutritional Healing</u> (2nd edition) by James F. Balch, M.D. and Phyllis A. Balch, C.N.C. Avery Publishing Group: Garden City Park, NY, 1997.

A helpful guide to herbal, vitamin, food, and other drug-free remedies and preventative treatments. Easy to read and informative—a must for anyone interested in holistic health.

14. <u>PDR for Herbal Medicines</u> (1st edition). Medical Economics Company: Montvale, NJ, 1998.

Everything you wanted to know about herbs—and more. This helpful guide lists chemical properties of herbs, history, habitat, what they're used for, side effects, etc. You may need to look up in a medical dictionary some of the medical terms.

15. <u>The American Medical Association Encyclopedia of Medicine</u>. Charles B. Clayman, M.D., Medical Editor. Random House: New York, 1989.

Do you want to know where the lymph nodes are? See how a CAT-scan works? Learn the difference between a harmless cold and spinal meningitis? This easy-to-use book comes with helpful illustrations and explanations of complicated conditions and medical terms—in everyday English. Everybody should have one. It's not for making your own diagnosis, but it can help you become a lot more informed about your body and the medical world.

16. <u>The Complete Cancer Survival Guide</u>. Peter Teeley and Philip Bashe. Doubleday: New York, 2000.

A comprehensive source book for all types and treatments of cancer. It's thick and full of information—the encyclopedia of cancer! Easy to read—a must for all cancer patients and their families.

17. <u>Dr. Susan Love's Breast Book</u>. Susan M. Love, M.D. with Karen Lindsey. Perseus Books: New York, 2000.

All you need to know about breasts, what can go wrong

with them, and how to keep them healthy. It has a good section on breast cancer, treatment, and prevention.

18. <u>Women's Health Companion</u>. Susan M. Lark, M.D. Celestial Arts Publishing: Berkeley, CA, 1995.

A general guide to women's health, including diet, lifestyle, exercise, etc.

19. <u>The Breast Cancer Prevention Diet</u>. Dr. Bob Arnot. Little, brown and Company: New York, 1998.

An easy-to-follow diet to help prevent breast cancer (eat the right fats, avoid sugar, and stock up on fresh vegetables!).

20. <u>It's Not About the Bike: My Journey Back to Life</u> by Lance Armstrong and Sally Jenkins, 2002.

The many-time Tour d'France winner candidly discusses his cancer and treatment, including medical procedures, workouts, and the road to recovery as a world-class athlete.

21. <u>Childhood Cancer Survivors: A Practical Guide to Your Future</u> by Nancy Keene and others, 2000.

The author gives much helpful information about the physical, emotional, psychological, and social aspects of cancer in young people. It includes a helpful section on the long-term effects of chemotherapy, and even a little book where you can keep information about the medications and other aspects of your treatment.

22. <u>Hannah's Gift: Lessons from a Life Fully Lived</u> by Maria Housden, 2002.

A mother chronicles the death of her three-year-old daughter to cancer. Little Hannah lived fully, dancing in her glittery red shoes in the hospital room. Hannah brought joy to all she touched. This book will bring comfort to anyone troubled by loss.

Books about Miscarriage or Surviving a Traumatic Experience

1. <u>Roses in December: Finding Strength Within Grief</u> by Marilyn Willett Heavilin, 1998.

A touching, simple, honest book about a mother's loss of a newborn, a baby to SIDS, and a teenage son to a drunk driver. Marilyn is a friend of mine, and she's a great speaker. She got involved with The Compassionate Friends (www.compassionatefriends.org), a grief support group for those who have lost children or who have had miscarriages. She helps people see God's love through grief.

2. <u>A Rose in Heaven</u> by Dawn Siegrist Waltman, 1999.

An uplifting, healing book that helps the reader through the grief process, written by a woman who lost her baby. Great for anyone who loses a child at any stage of pregnancy or after birth. It goes from sorrow to a peace of knowing that God has a plan for everybody. It has a memory idea section to help a mother remember her lost child. The last entry, "Joy in the Morning," brings hope.

3. <u>Miscarriage: Why it Happens and How Best to Reduce Your Risks—A Doctor's Guide to the Facts</u> by Henry Lerner, M.D. and others, 2003.

Dr. Lerner has compiled the most current medical information about the causes of miscarriage, diagnostic tests, and medical procedures. He also deals with the emotional and psychological aspects.

4. <u>Empty Cradle, Broken Heart: Surviving the Death of Your Baby</u> by Deborah L. Davis, ph.D., 1996.

The author uses quotes and stories from bereaved parents to encourage those who have lost a baby. She gently explores the medical, social, and emotional processes and helps grieving parents examine their grief because they are not alone. She has a section just for fathers and a section on how to enjoy your living children without being overprotective.

5. <u>Miscarriage: A Woman Doctor's Story</u> by Lynn Friedman and Irene Daria, 2001.

Dr. Lynn Friedman helps you get through miscarriage with her wisdom, support, and experience as an obstetrician. She tackles the question of "why" and offers facts about how to try and prevent future miscarriages, the use of medical procedures, grief therapy, a section on "trying again," and 3 women's stories.

6. <u>A Silent Love: Personal Stories of Coming to Terms with Miscarriage</u> by Adrienne Ryan, 2001.

The author, who suffered multiple miscarriages, urges miscarriage, stillbirth, or neonatal death sufferers to talk about their experience and so help them cope with their grief. She explains why this type of grief is unique and has a collection of over 50 real-life stories by mothers, fathers, and grandparents.

7. <u>When a Baby Dies: A Handbook for Healing and Helping</u> by Rana K. Limbo and others, 1998.

The book covers individual stories of pregnancy and perinatal loss, with chapters of miscarriage, ectopic pregnancy, stillbirth, newborn death, and loss in a multiple gestation pregnancy. The book addresses family issues that occur as each person grieves differently. It also includes helpful medical information and checklists.

8. Help, Comfort and Hope After Losing Your Baby in Pregnancy or the First Year by Hannah Lothrop, 1997.

Lothrop offers grieving parents comforting, practical advice about how to cope with their loss. This information can help medical and other caregivers understand how parents feel. Lothrop uses her first-hand knowledge and empathy to guide bereaved parents in their grieving process that resolves grief into acceptance.

9. All Rivers Run to the Sea: Memoirs by Elie Weisel and Jon Rothschild, 1995.

Autobiography of the 1986 Nobel Peace Prize for Literature winner. He discusses his early life as a young Jewish scholar and teenager in concentration camps—and life after liberation.

10. And the Sea is Never Full: Memoirs by Elie Weisel and Miriam Weisel. 1999.

The sequel to his first autobiography, about his life as an activist and journalist and how he won the Nobel Peace Prize.

11. Night by Elie Weisel and others, 1982.

One of the greatest memoirs of the Holocaust, written like a novel from a teenager's point of view.

Some of my Favorite Books

1. The Bible (I like the New King James version).

2. Anything by C.S. Lewis, especially:

<u>The Chronicles of Narnia</u> (his children's fantasy stories, set of 7).
<u>Out of the Silent Planet</u>; <u>Perelandria</u>; and <u>That Hideous Strength</u>
(his science fiction trilogy).
<u>Mere Christianity</u> (his theology).
<u>A Grief Observed</u> (the journal of his wife's cancer and death).
<u>The Problem of Pain</u> (taking on that tough topic of why God allows us to suffer).
<u>The Great Divorce</u> (a sort of modern <u>Paradise Lost</u>).
<u>The Screwtape Letters</u> (letters from one demon to another on how to trip up Christians; very insightful and imaginative).
<u>Surprised by Joy</u> (Lewis' autobiography of his early life as an atheist and scholar and how he became a Christian).

3. Anything by J.R.R. Tolkien, especially:

<u>The Hobbit</u> (the story of Bilbo Baggins and his adventure in finding The Ring).
<u>The Lord of the Rings</u> trilogy (<u>The Fellowship of the Ring</u>;

The Two Towers; and The Return of the King)—need I say anything?
The Silmarillion (the early history of Middle-earth).
The Letters of J.R.R. Tolkien (letters he wrote to friends and family).

4. J.R.R. Tolkien: A Biography by Humphrey Carpenter (the only authorized biography of Tolkien, by a close friend).

5. Finding God in The Lord of the Rings by Kurt Bruner and Jim Ware (two Christians look at the Christian symbolism, etc. in Tolkien's work).

6. The Lord of the Rings Official Movie Guide by Brian Sibley (great pictures of New Zealand remote locations, sets, costumes, and swords—along with interviews of the director, artistic director, actors, etc.).

7. The Fairie Queen by Edmund Spencer (English Renaissance at its best—beautiful poetry about a romance between the fairie queen and her knight).

8. The complete works of William Shakespeare (What can I say? The Bard knew how to use words. My favorite plays are Hamlet and Richard II).

9. Paradise Lost by John Milton (the saga of Adam and Eve in poetic form).

10. Poems and essays by John Donne (the blind 17th Century poet writes some really cool ideas).

11. Romantic Poets of the 17th and 18th Century: William Blake, Robert Burns, Sir Walter Scott, Samuel Taylor Coleridge, Mary Wordsworth, Percy Bysshe Shelley, John Keats, Lord Byron, and Edgar Allen Poe.

12. Poems by Alfred, Lord Tennyson.

13. Poems by Robert Browning and Elizabeth Barrett Browning.

14. <u>A Tale of Two Cities</u> by Charles Dickens (a riveting story of love, betrayal, and self-sacrifice during the French Revolution).

15. Poems by Emily Dickinson.

16. Poems by Robert Frost.

17. <u>The Tale of King Arthur and the Knights of the Round Table</u> by Sir Thomas Mallory (the old-fashioned version of Camelot).

18. <u>Fairy Tales</u> by Hans Christian Anderson (a misfit himself, Hans wrote stories that often had unhappy endings but taught great lessons).

19. <u>Heidi</u> by Johanna Spyri (set in the Swiss Alps, about an orphaned girl and her grandfather).

20. The <u>Little House</u> series (set of 9 books) by Laura Ingalls Wilder (Laura tells her story of growing up on the American Prairie in the 1800s, with honesty, details, and simplicity).

21. <u>The Princess and the Goblin</u> by George MacDonald (the 18th Century Scottish pastor creates a rich fantasy about an underground horde of goblins about to take over the princess' castle. The princess gets help from a lowly miner boy—and her mysterious grandmother).

22. <u>Alice in Wonderland</u> by Lewis Carroll (When Alice fell down that rabbit hole, all sorts of amazing things began to

happen. This book helped spark a world of fantasy stories for children).

23. The Adventures of Huckleberry Finn by Mark Twain (this tale of a boy's journey down the Mississippi River in the 1800s is richly described, with the humor and wit we would expect from Mark Twain).

24. Madeleine L'Engle's science fiction books: A Wrinkle in Time; A Wind in the Door; A Swiftly Tilting Planet; Many Waters; and An Acceptable Time (the Christian daughter of a scientist mixes physics with fantasy, courage, and love as brothers and sisters explore the universe. The first book won the Newberry Award for Best Children's Book of the Year).

25. The Bronze Bow by Elizabeth George Speare (a Roman meets Jesus and learns that Romans and Jews can love each other—another Newberry Award Winner).

26. Island of the Blue Dolphins by Scott O'Dell (another Newberry Award Winner about a girl left alone on a Pacific island, and how she survives and learns to love the natural world and its creatures).

27. The Sword of Shannara by Terry Brooks (high fantasy in a strange land populated by interesting creatures and, especially, elves. Thanks, Terry—your book sparked me to write my first fantasy novel).

28. The Giving Tree by Shel Silverstein (a classic children's book about a tree who just wants to give to an unappreciative boy).

29. The Ann of Green Gables series by Lucy Maud Montgomery (how much trouble can a young orphan, who gets

adopted by an older brother and sister on a beautiful Canadian Island at the turn of the 20th Century, get into?).

DVDs, Videos, and Music CDs

1. <u>Living with Cancer: A Message of Hope</u> VHS video by Wellspring Media, 2000.

Narrated by Anne Bancroft, this video has cancer patients and professionals discuss the disease and how they survived. It even has jokes by a cancer surviving comedian.

2. <u>Between Us</u> VHS video by Mary Katzke, 1998.

A support group for women with breast cancer. Survivors share their stories.

3. <u>No Hair Day: Laughing (and Crying) Our Way Through Breast Cancer</u> VHS video by WGBH Boston, 2001.

Three breast cancer patients share their own stories of treatment, wigs, and emotions. They show how cancer isn't always frowning.

4. <u>Harry Potter: Witchcraft Repackaged</u> VHS video by Loyal Publishing, 2001.

A documentary look at the Harry Potter phenomenon, its use of real witchcraft items, and how it has increased interest in modern-day witchcraft, witchcraft books, and witchcraft websites.

5. The Lord of the Rings trilogy: The Fellowship of the Ring (2001); The The Towers (2002); and The Return of the King (2003), VHS or DVD by New Line Cinema.

Tolkien's saga is brought to the big screen with beautiful cinematography of New Zealand's natural wonders; costume, prop, and set amazements; and a host of fine actors such as Elijah Wood as Frodo, Sean Austin as Samwise, Ian McKellen as Gandalf, Viggo Mortensen as Aragorn, Liv Tyler as Arwen, and Cate Blanchett as Galadriel. Directed by Kiwi Peter Jackson who shows us that a great film doesn't have to be made by Hollywood. Academy Award-winners. PG-13.

6. Alien (1979) and Aliens (1986) VHS or DVDs by 20th Century Fox.

Not for the faint of heart, these science fiction/horror movies show how crewmember Ripley (Sigourney Weaver) battles aliens—and what it can be like to battle cancer. Directed by Ridley Scott. R.

7. Ladyhawk (1985) VHS or DVD by 20th Century Fox.

Medieval Knights at their best as Rutger Hauer, with his huge black horse, big sword, and pet hawk, tries to end the enchantment that separates him from his love, Michelle Pfeiffer. Matthew Broderick is the comic thief who unexpectedly helps them, along with an alcoholic priest played by Leo McKern. John Wood is the heartless bad bishop who enchanted the couple. Great cinematography, shot in Europe, with real castles. Directed by Richard Donner. PG-13.

8. First Knight (1995) VHS or DVD by Columbia Pictures.

King Arthur (Sean Connery) and Guinevere (Julia Ormond) get their lives complicated and helped by unconventional knight Lancelot (Richard Gere) as they battle the evil Malagant (played convincingly by Ben Cross). In this version, Lancelot and Guinevere resist temptation pretty well. Great Christian message and symbolism, with beautiful English/Scottish castles and settings. Directed by Jerry Zucker. Rated PG-13.

9. Quo Vadis (1951) VHS by MGM.

An epic like they don't make them anymore, this film tells the story of a Roman General (Robert Taylor) who falls in love with a Christian slave (Deborah Kerr) during the First Century. Emperor Nero (Peter Ustinov, won an Oscar for his role) soon has Rome burning and blames it on the Christians. This starts a great persecution with the young couple fighting wild animals in the arena. Academy Award for Best Picture. Directed by Mervyn LeRoy. Not Rated.

10. The Robe (1953) VHS by 20th Century Fox.

Richard Burton stars as the Roman centurion Marcellus who crucified Jesus and inherited The Robe. Jean Simmons is his Roman girlfriend who later becomes a Christian. Victor Mature is the slave who helps Marcellus understand Christ's love, resurrection, and forgiveness. Academy Award-winner. Directed by Henry Koster. Not Rated.

11. Ben-Hur (1959) VHS by MGM.

Another epic (with 500,00 extras and 15,000 in the chariot race), this film starts in Israel during the Roman occupation and the time of Jesus' ministry. Ben-Hur, a Judean Prince (Charlton Heston won an Oscar for this role) is arrested by his boyhood friend, a Roman turned soldier (Jack Hawkins). Hur's mother and sister are imprisoned while Hur is sent off as a galley slave to Rome. Along the way, Jesus gives the thirsty prisoner some water, and Hur looks into eyes he will never forget. After escaping the galley and rescuing a Roman General, Hur is adopted and becomes a Roman citizen and chariot-racer. But he cannot forget his mother, sister, and the Jewish girl who loves him. He returns to Israel bent on revenge against the Roman who imprisoned them. But his great hatred turns to love when he meets Jesus on Crucifixion Day. Academy Award for Best Picture. Directed by Karl Tunberg. G.

12. <u>Matthew</u> (1997) VHS by The Visual Bible.

A 4-video set, this series plays out the Gospel of Matthew, with believable acting, authentic setting, and period costumes. The screenplay is word for word from the Bible. Starring Richard Kiley as Matthew and Bruce Marchiano as Jesus. Great for showing children or anyone who wants to see the Gospel brought to life onscreen. Directed by Regardt Van Den Bergh. Not Rated. Check out their website at www.visualbible.com.

13. <u>Acts</u> (1997) VHS by The Visual Bible.

This 4-video set tells the story of the First Century Church after the Resurrection of Jesus, from the amazing event of Pentecost to persecution, to the long journeys of spreading the Gospel to Asia Minor, Greece, and Rome—with miracles, narrow escapes, martyrs, and great adventures. Dean Jones is Luke, the narrator. James Brolin plays Peter the Apostle, and Henry O. Arnold is Saul the Jewish Persecutor who gets blinded by the light and becomes Paul, who wrote much of the New Testament and spread the Gospel all the way to Rome. Directed by Regardt Van Den Bergh. Not Rated. Check out their website at www.visualbible.com.

14. <u>Speechless</u> (1999) Music CD by Sparrow Records.

Incredibly moving songs by singer/songwriter/musician Steven Curtis Chapman. Includes my all-time favorite "Dive" (about diving into the Living River). Also includes "Great Expectations," "Fingerprints of God," "The Invitation," "The Change," and the humorous "Whatever." A mix of fast, cutting-edge, experimental, and slow music, including a memorial called "With Hope," about the loss of a child. It ends with a sweet song called "Be Still and Know."

15. Declaration (2001) Music DC by Sparrow Records.

The sequel to Speechless, a faster, more lively collection that starts with "Live Out Loud" and "Jesus is Life." It slows down for "God is God" (a song that questions grief) and "When Love Takes You In" (a song about adopting children). "No Greater Love" uses Amazon Indian music and a native song by Mincaye, an Indian who toured with Chapman. This CD is cutting-edge, experimental, and ballad-like in its variety.

Interview with My Husband, Edd Williams

July 15, 2003
(I've done interviews with top figure skaters, pastors, and others, and this was one of the best)

Lonna: What are your thoughts about your wife having survived cancer?

Edd: Well, I'm obviously very satisfied and happy that she survived cancer. I mean, if you don't survive cancer, you die. And it's been seven years. Faced with that type of a trial, at the time it was very challenging because we were put to the ultimate test as to how much we really trusted the Lord Jesus and how much we were willing to surrender to Him in order to put ourselves completely and utterly dependent on Him. I'm delighted that it was in the Lord's will to have her survive. Surviving cancer causes you to appreciate every single day that you have and to think more and more about what could have happened. It's sort of like a near miss with a bullet or a traffic accident. You suddenly realize how vulnerable and frail you are. When a person survives that sort of thing, you walk away from it a lot more appreciative of life and what you have.

Lonna: What helped you get through the whole cancer experience?

Edd: It came down to a very significant moment in time when I was working in the yard down in the valley, and I was discing the property with the tractor. I think by that time Lonna had had her second or third chemo treatment. She was real sick, and there were a couple of women (from the church) in our house, and I was out in the yard, and it was hot. I felt the Holy Spirit come over me, and I was afraid and concerned and hopeful and all those things. When the Holy Spirit fell on me, I dropped off the tractor and landed on my knees on the soft dirt that I'd already disced and said, "God, if it's Your will that she passes away, then that's OK. And if it's Your will that she survive, that's OK. I was at a place of total surrender. Then the Holy Spirit convinced me in my heart that Lonna was going to survive. That's where I got my confidence during the rest of her treatments to be optimistic about her prognosis and the outcome.

Lonna: What's it been like having small children through the whole ordeal, and also the recovery period during the last seven years after the end of the chemo treatments?

Edd: Well, with the little kids it was scary because I thought, what if Lonna did pass away? Then the children would be without a mom. If Lonna died the year after treatment, then Jonathan would have been only two and Jessie about five. I would have been a widower with two very small babies, and it would have been tough to be a single dad. I would have been miserably brokenhearted. It would have been difficult. In terms of the recovery period, it was me doing more around the house and helping with the kids and just trying to be a servant in as many ways as I could without killing myself. Remember that I had three jobs at the time, and it was difficult. I was driving five or six hundred miles a week, teaching at three different districts, seven or eight classes. It was a really difficult time.

Lonna: How do you think your quality of life is now, seven years after chemo?

Edd: A lot of things have happened since Lonna and I both got to that place of total surrender. I think God has honored that. I think God gave me the job that I have. There were over 200 qualified applicants for that job. That has allowed Lonna to stay home and homeschool. God has graciously given me different types of ministries including a lot of music ministry, and I think all of these are the fruits of our faith. I'd like to think that our faith was part of the healing factor for Lonna, but I believe in a sovereign God, so the decision for Lonna not to die was God's decision, not ours, but it was our hope. I think the quality of life has increased tremendously because we appreciate each other and what we have more. God has richly blessed us with a good-paying job, our children are homeschooled, we're living in a beautiful place, in an extraordinarily beautiful home. If I didn't know any better, I would say that our life is abundantly comfortable, and that is probably not a good place for Christians to be in.

Lonna: So how do you think the whole cancer experience affected the young children, Jessica and Jonathan?

Edd: I think Jonathan was too young for it to affect him one way or the other except that he had to stop breastfeeding earlier than he wanted to. Jessica was old enough, I think, to sense that something was wrong, and now that she has grown through these seven years and she's almost eleven years old, she has become more acutely aware of what cancer is and how it could have taken her mother from her. So I think Jessie directly is more tender-hearted and more appreciative of life and maybe even more melancholy sometimes because she empathizes with people who are in pain. Jonathan, I think, has borrowed from her and watched her and listened to what we have to say about how his mother went through chemo and is probably a little bit scared and concerned about the future because of this cancer thing. So I think the kids are hypersensitive to their loved ones and empathetic towards others—more so than most children.

Lonna: And what about you? Have you changed because of the cancer?

Edd: The cancer caused me personally to grow much more quickly in my willingness to surrender everything to the Lord. So in that respect the cancer spurred me in a much faster pace in my Christian growth. It helped me to evaluate my attitudes about materialism, things, my relationship with Lonna. It helped me to appreciate life more and material things less because they are less important, obviously. A person becomes much more in tune with that attitude when the possibility of death is right in your face. I love my children more as a result of it because I view life as precious and frail and that it can disappear quickly, anytime. We saw many people die who had cancer, in the various groups we came in contact with, like visiting City of Hope and going to those chemo treatments and seeing the people who were without hair and dying. It was difficult because then you become very much aware of how quickly life can go away.

Lonna: How do you think having gone through five miscarriages has affected you?

Edd: That is collectively the most difficult thing of all. I really ache sometimes when I think about the children we might have had. In particular that one miscarriage in December of 1997 when the baby was completely formed and was a little boy. Lonna gave birth to him in our bedroom and then I took him outside and buried him in our yard. We named him Michael. Before I buried him I looked at him closely and I studied him, and I could see how much he would look like Jonathan if he would have grown up. When I look at Jonathan I sometimes think about the children we haven't had. I don't get depressed about it because I really appreciate the two children we do have. I might be more depressed if we didn't have any children.

Sometimes I wonder what it would be like if we had more kids. I know it would be harder in terms of finances and logistics, but I think I would like to have more than the two that we have. I love the two that we have, don't get me wrong.

Lonna: Do you appreciate them more?

Edd: Yeah, I do. I even appreciate other people's kids more.

Lonna: Do you think you're more overprotective of them because of those miscarriages?

Edd: No, I wouldn't say that. I think whether or not we had two or five children, I'd behave pretty much the same way. Children need to be protected. They need to be warned about potential hazards. I think parents who just let their kids run off are not being very good parents.

Lonna: What do you think about your wife writing her story about all that—the cancer and miscarriages?

Edd: Well, I think there are two sides to this coin. There is the one side that could serve to help others. Then there's another side that could serve to be therapeutic to the writer. I know that when I write there is a lot of therapy when I ventilate my feelings and experiences on the page. If I were reading a book by an author I didn't know, and that author talked almost exclusively about him or herself, and then I felt like the material was just therapeutic and didn't have a connection with audience, I don't think I would be very happy about that. I think a project is justified and should be written and published if it is motivated by ministry. I think if its' motivated by the individual and her interest in herself—the writer sort of imploding—I don't know if I would consider that glorifying God.

Lonna: If you felt that the author were trying to share her story to bring people to Christ through difficult times—

Edd: That's a whole different ballgame. It's sort of like when a preacher gets up and talks about himself the whole time. If those examples don't have anything to do with the Scripture that he's talking about, he should keep his mouth shut. But if those examples make more concrete the ideas in the Scripture that he's preaching on, then by all means—because that preacher is using his own experience to reach people. I've heard preachers talk about themselves, and I don't get the connection between what they're preaching on and what they're talking about. To me that's just self indulgence, and I don't think it brings glory to Christ.

Lonna: And if the writing is full of Scripture—

Edd: There's power in the Word. There may be emotional power, and it can have an affect on people and a happy ending if it's self-indulgent, because M.L. Rosenthal said that our experience is connected to the common life. It's that common life that our confessional stories touch, and other people can relate. But when the Word is connected to the story, the power is in the Word and not in the story. So if somebody is going to write a book about what they went through—no matter what it is, child abuse or divorce or anger management or cancer—whatever it is, as long as it is connected to ministry and outreach, witnessing about the wonderful Lord that we have, then I think it is a good thing.

Lonna: So you agree with your wife putting in a lot of Scripture because you believe as she does that those words are Life and Real and life-changing?

Edd: Isaiah 55:11 says that "My Word shall not return to Me void." If we use His Word, God will use writing to serve His own ends and purposes. If we use our own words, I think they are essentially dead without God's Spirit behind them.

Lonna: So you write music sometimes and play music and lead worship. How do you feel about that?

Edd: When I write music—at least the last ten years this has been true—I pray before, during, and after because I don't want what I write to be mine. I want it to be God's, and I want it to bring glory to Him and not to myself. I think it's the same thing with leading worship. A worship leader can get up there and be kind of prideful and cocky and high-minded and be very talented and sing up a storm and play three instruments and walk off stage and go outside and shake hands with people who all say "you did a wonderful job today." And it's all you, you, you instead of Jesus, Jesus, Jesus. That same person, if his heart is in the right place, can get up there and play three instruments and lead worship and not really draw attention to himself because he is seeking the Holy Spirit's power, and he's even saying he wants all the attention to go to Jesus. So worship leaders have to be very careful. So do writers. If they're motivated by self interest, I know that doesn't bring glory to God. If they're motivated by their relationship to Jesus and their desire to tell people about Jesus and how Jesus has affected their lives and even healed their lives, then by all means, talk. But keep the power of the Word in there and the attention on Jesus and not yourself.

Lonna: What do you think about your wife giving away her books?

Edd: I think that should take place. We don't often get paid for witnessing. Sometimes we pay a price to witness, just like missionaries who might pay thousands of dollars to get to that place where they serve the Lord and to stay there. Ultimately it all comes back to God; it's all for God. If you're spending seven dollars a book or whatever it costs you and giving that away, that's ministry. Ministry isn't free. So giving away the books is a good thing, depending on how your heart feels and the Holy Spirit is instructing you.

Lonna: Is there anything else you'd like to add about all this?

Edd: Well, I have a couple things. First, when a person within the family is diagnosed with cancer, it's very easy to focus on the cancer and to focus on what the cancer might do and to forget that cancer is only one of the ways that we can die. There's no guarantee. Sometimes we can put our energies too much on one thing and pray too much about one thing and forget about the others. In my case, as the husband, I was praying earnestly for my wife, but I could easily forget to pray for my friends, my children, and everything else because I'm putting too much attention on one thing. I could easily have died in a car accident or some other event that would have caused me to die first. Just because someone is diagnosed with cancer does not mean that everybody else in the family is OK.

Second, just because a person is in remission doesn't mean that the cancer isn't going to come back. So seven years later you think to yourself, great, she's healed, there are no traces of cancer in her body that doctors can find in her blood or any test. One of my colleagues, John Biehl, was married to Linda. She was cancer-free for ten years, and she then she got cancer and within two years was dead. I know other people who were in remission for five years, eight years, ten years—some more than that—and they got cancer again. So, the one side of the coin is that just because one member of the family has cancer doesn't mean that all of us are somehow immune to dying. The other side is that just because that person is apparently cured doesn't mean that the cancer can't come back. So those two things combined cause me to be a lot more aware of my day-to-day life and appreciative of my day-to-day life. The Scripture says "This is the day the Lord has made; I will rejoice and be glad in it." That Scripture is pointing to a very important principle: every single day is a gift from God and precious, and we should take advantage of that. Psalm 90:12 says "So teach me to number my days that I may pursue wisdom." We don't have all that much time. Our life is but a vapor, and it is gone. So why should we waste our time while we're here? Instead, we should be numbering our days, seeking the Lord every day, and growing in the knowledge of Him, earnestly, because we don't have any guarantees of how long we're going to be here.

ABOUT THE AUTHOR

Lonna Lisa Williams has been writing since the age of four. She went on to college and received a Master's degree in English, then taught college for 10 years. She has published poetry in a variety of literary magazines. "Like a Tree Planted," an environmental science fiction novel, was her first book. "Selah of the Summit," her fantasy novel, is a Christian alternative to "Harry Potter" and the first book in a trilogy. "Crossing the Chemo Room," her second book, is Lonna's true, inspirational cancer survival story. "I Saw You in the Moon" is its long-awaited sequel. All of Lonna's books are published by GreatUnpublished.com.

After her husband Edd got a full-time job as an English professor, Lonna gave up teaching college English to stay home and raise her children. She lives with her family in the California mountains where she enjoys writing, photography, hiking, and figure skating. You can visit her website at www.lonnawilliams.com.

ABOUT GREATUNPUBLISHED.COM

www.greatunpublished.com is a website that exists to serve writers and readers, and to remove some of the commercial barriers between them. When you purchase a GreatUNpublished title, whether you order it in electronic form or in a paperback volume, the author is receiving a majority of the post-production revenue.

A GreatUNpublished book is never out of stock, and always available, because each book is printed on-demand, as it is ordered.

A portion of the site's share of profits is channeled into literacy programs.

So by purchasing this title from GreatUNpublished, you are helping to revolutionize the publishing industry for the benefit of writers and readers.

And for this we thank you.